Air Fryer Cookbook

For Beginners In 2020

Easy, Healthy And Delicious Recipes

For A Nourishing Meal

(Includes Index, Some Low Carb Recipes, Air Fryer FAQs

And Troubleshooting Tips)

By

Barbara Trisler

www.MillenniumPublishingLimited.com

Copyright ©2020

Disclaimer

This publication is designed to provide competent and reliable information regarding the subject matter covered. However, it is sold with the understanding that the author is not engaged in rendering medical or other professional advice. Laws and practices often vary from state to state and country to country and if medical or other expert assistance is required, the services of a professional should be sought. The author specifically disclaims any liability that is incurred from the use or application of the contents of this book.

Table of Contents

What Is This Book All About?

This book contains proven steps and strategies on how to start preparing healthy and delicious meals that you can serve any time of the day using only one appliance – *the Air Fryer*. This innovation makes it possible to enjoy fried foods with less oil. You can also use it to whip up a wide range of dishes, snacks, and desserts.

It features loads of recipes that you can tweak in many ways to suit your preference and the availability of ingredients. Each recipe has a nutrient content guide per serving. In addition, it explains the basics about the appliance and the benefits of using it as compared to the traditional manner of frying food.

Finally, it also contains a quick guide of measurement conversion that can become handy when preparing your ingredients.

Please Note - There are two different version of this book – one with pictures and another without pictures. This particular version has *no pictures*. This is because of the prohibitive cost of printing images in color.

However, do not worry. A bonus PDF image booklet is available for download. It shows each recipe in this book in full color. See the end of this book for details on how to get it.

Without further ado, lets get started!

What is An Air Fryer?

An air fryer utilizes the convection mechanism in cooking food. It circulates hot air through the use of a mechanical fan to cook the ingredients inside the fryer. **The process eliminates the use of too much oil** in the traditional way of frying but still cooks food via the Maillard effect (i.e. a chemical reaction between an amino acid and a reducing sugar, usually requiring the addition of heat).

The process was named after the person who first explained it in 1912, French chemist Louis-Camille Maillard. The effect gives a distinctive flavor to browned foods, such as bread, biscuits, cookies, pan-fried meat, seared steaks, and many more.

The air fryer requires only a thin layer of oil for the ingredients to cook. It circulates hot air up to 392 degrees Fahrenheit. It's an innovative way of eliminating up to 80 percent of the oil that is traditionally used to fry different foods and prepare pastries.

You can find a dose of friendly features in air fryers depending on the brand you're using. Most brands include a timer adjustment and temperature control setting to make cooking easier and precise. An air fryer comes with a cooking basket where you'll place the food. The basket is placed on top of a drip tray. Depending on the model you're using, you will either be prompted to shake the basket to distribute oil evenly or it automatically does the job via a food agitator.

This is perfect for home use but if you're cooking for many people and you want to apply the same cooking technique, you can put your food items in specialized air crisper trays and cook them using a convection oven. An air fryer and convection oven apply the same technique in cooking but an air fryer has a smaller build and produces less heat.

How to Use Your Air Fryer

This appliance comes with a manual for easy assembly and as a handy guide for first-time users. Most brands also include a pamphlet of recipes to give you ideas about the wide range of dishes that you can create using this single kitchen appliance. Once you are ready to cook and you have all your ingredients ready, put them in the basket and insert it into the fryer. Other recipes will require you to preheat the air fryer before using. Once the basket is in, set the temperature and timer and begin cooking.

You can use an air fryer to cook food in a variety of ways. Once you get used with the basics, you can try its other features, such as advanced baking and using air fryer dehydrators.

Here are some of the cooking techniques that you can do with this single appliance:

- **Fry**: You can actually omit oil in cooking but a little amount adds crunch and flavor to your food. You can add oil to the ingredients while mixing or lightly spray the food with oil before cooking. You can use most kinds of oils but many users prefer peanut, olive, sunflower, and canola oils.
- **Roast**: You can produce the same quality of roasted foods like the ones cooked in a conventional roaster in a faster manner. This is recommended to people who need to come up with a special dish but do not have much time to prepare.
- **Bake**: There are baking pans suited for this appliance that you can use to bake bread, cookies, and other pastries. It only takes around 15 to 30 minutes to get your baked goodies done.

- **Grill**: It effectively grills your food easily and without mess. You only need to shake the basket halfway through the cooking process or flip the ingredients once or twice depending on the instructions. To make it easier, you can put the ingredients in a grill pan or grill layer with a handle, which other models include in the package or you can also buy one as an added accessory.

There are many kinds of foods that you can cook using an air fryer, but there are also certain types that are not suited for it. Avoid cooking ingredients, which can be steamed, like beans and carrots. You also cannot fry foods covered in heavy batter in this appliance.

Aside from the above mentioned, you can cook most kinds of ingredients using an air fryer. You can use it to cook foods covered in light flour or bread crumbs. You can cook a variety of vegetables in the appliance, such as cauliflower, asparagus, zucchini, kale, peppers, and corn on the cob. You can also use it to cook frozen foods and home prepared meals by following a different set of instructions for these purposes.

An air fryer also comes with another useful feature - the separator. It allows you to cook multiple dishes at a time. Use the separator to divide ingredients in the pan or basket. You have to make sure that all ingredients have the same temperature setting so that everything will cook evenly at the same time.

The Benefits of Air fryer

It is important to note that air fried foods are still fried. Unless you've decided to eliminate the use of oils in cooking, you must still be cautious about the food you eat. Despite that, it clearly presents a better and healthier option than deep frying. It helps you avoid unnecessary fats and oils, which makes it an ideal companion when you intend to lose weight. It offers a lot more benefits, which include the following:

- It is convenient and easy to use, plus, it's easy to clean.
- It doesn't give off unwanted smells when cooking.
- You can use it to prepare a variety of meals.
- It can withstand heavy cooking.
- It is durable and made of metal and high-grade plastic.
- Cooking using this appliance is not as messy as frying in a traditional way. You don't have to worry about greasy spills and stains in the kitchen.

Air Fryer Troubleshooting Tips

No matter the brand or how expensive an air fryer is, you are still bound to experience certain technical problems caused either by regular wear-and-tear or damages due to mishandling. You also cannot always foresee or prevent accidents in the kitchen, which can cause parts of the air fryer to malfunction.

Regardless of the cause, it is important for you to learn how to analyze and solve these technical issues if you own an air fryer—or even if you're yet to purchase one. Here are the common problems encountered before, during, and after cooking with an air fryer:

Problem #1

The air fryer is not turning on despite being plugged into a power source, or it suddenly loses power in the middle of cooking.

The best way to address this issue is to eliminate one by one the probable causes until you have reached the most likely root of this problem.

In this particular case, check first if the air fryer would turn on if you plug it in to another electric socket. If you are using an extension cord for this, discontinue such practice because the machine has high power requirements that may be outside the capacity of your extension cord. It is also a fire hazard since the extension itself may overheat and burst into flames when it is used inappropriately.

There are some models that do not turn on unless the basket is placed properly. Remove the basket and then return it carefully. Pay close attention on how well the basket is fitted with the rest of air fryer.

If the air fryer still doesn't turn on, inspect the power cord of the machine itself. Check if there are any deep and visible cuts or other types of damages to the wires by running through your gaze and fingers along the cord. When doing so, it is best to first unplug the air fryer to avoid being electrocuted.

If you have found signs of damage, then it might be the cause for this power issue. This is not likely to be covered by the machine's warranty, unless the air fryer has just been purchased and never been used before. Otherwise, you would have to pay a capable technician to replace the damaged power cord of your air fryer.

In case that there is no damage, check if another equipment would work when it is plugged into the power sockets that you have tried earlier. If the other equipment works, then the problem lies with the air fryer itself. Bring it to the nearest service center, or call a technician to repair it for a fee. However, if the problem is with the socket, then ask an electrician to handle the problem with the wiring or fuse box instead.

Problem #2

A stream of white smoke is coming out of the top and sides of the air fryer.

Do not be alarmed yet since white smoke can mean either of these two things when it comes to air frying. First, that smoke might actually be steam from the food being cooked inside. If it smells similar to the food itself or how you expect the food to smell like when it is cooked, then there is nothing to worry about.

The other possible cause for the white smoke is an electrical problem. Check if the smoke smells like burning plastic or rubber. That is a bad sign, and you should take immediate action. Unplug the air fryer, and call an electrician as soon as possible.

Problem #3

The air fryer is emitting black smoke in the middle of cooking.

Black smoke typically originates from the accumulated grease inside the air fryer. When you cook foods that contain high levels of fat without proper preparation, the fats would liquefy under high temperatures and would then drip down the bottom of the air fryer basket. As the process of cooking continues, the grease would start to burn, emitting foul odors and black smoke.

To prevent the occurrence of black smoke whenever you fry fatty food, you can simply add a cup of water in the bottom part of the basket. By doing this, the melted fat would drip down into the water instead of directly on the basket. The grease would not burn while you are cooking, and as an added bonus, the air fryer would be easier to clean afterwards.

Problem #4
A cloud of blue smoke suddenly forms around the air fryer.

You must act quickly when this happens because blue smoke indicates severe electrical problems in either your socket or the air fryer itself. Usually, the appearance of blue smoke would be immediately followed by fire, so you have to address this problem as quickly as possible.

The first thing to do is unplug the air fryer. If fire has already started, use a fire extinguisher designed for electrical fires to put out the flames. Cut off the power in the circuit breaker, if you have access to it.

Even if there is no visible damage to the air fryer, do not use it until it has been checked by technicians or you have brought it to the service center. You might be advised to change some parts of the air fryer, or to buy a new one instead. Either way, you must have it checked before using it again since neglecting to do so would result to another electrical issue inside the kitchen.

Remember, using the air fryer without reading the instructions and reminders would definitely lead to technical difficulties later on. Failing to do so could not only cause you unnecessary expenses, but it could also be a threat to your safety and those around you.

Learning how to handle minor problems on your own can save you from having to pay technicians in order to get the air fryer back into its optimal condition. However, if you have done everything to address the issues of your air fryer, but the problem still persists, then it is advisable for you to consult experts at this point. Air fryers are complex machines, so do not attempt to troubleshoot major mechanical issues with what knowledge you have about similar equipment.

If the warranty period for your air fryer is still in effect, do not hesitate to refer your problem to the service center. The manufacturers and distributors have the obligation to sustain customer satisfaction, especially after the equipment has already been purchased. If the warranty period is over, then you may opt to take the fryer to an authorized service center instead. Do not rely on cheap repair shops since your air fryer might end up being damaged even further.

Save yourself from stress and additional expenses by letting trained experts handle the issues of your air fryer.

Frequently Asked Questions
If you have just purchased an air fryer or if you are still considering it, here are the most frequently asked questions about this fascinating kitchen equipment:

Question #1
Which types of food can be cooked using an air fryer?

The air fryer is capable of cooking or baking almost any type of food. It is not limited to just frying, despite its name. Depending on the model you have, an air fryer can be used to roast and grill meats and vegetables, as well bake certain types of breads and pastries.

For vegetables, there are some types that would yield better results when cooked with an air fryer. These include potatoes, corn, mushrooms, and zucchini. Natural vegetable chips are also great with air fryers. On the other hand, vegetables that are best served steamed or boiled are not suitable for air fryers.

Items that have been frozen may be cooked in an air fryer without having to thaw them out first. In fact, anything that can be cooked using an oven might be fried, grilled, roasted, or baked with the use of an air fryer.

Question #2
How much food can be cooked per batch?

This depends on the size and capacity of the air fryer. However, it is not recommended to fill up the air fryer basket to its full capacity since this will restrict the movement of hot air inside. This can then result to unevenly cooked food.

At most, the basket should only be half-filled per batch. Given this, an average sized air fryer can accommodate around two to three servings. You should also refer to the manual and the accompanying recipe book of the model that you have. These usually indicate the recommended batch sizes for each type of food that you can cook or bake.

It might be better as well to go for smaller batches while you are still trying to get acquainted with your air fryer. Observe how fast and how well the food has been cooked. If you were successful, then you can try going for bigger batches the next time you decide to cook that dish again.

Question #3
Does air fried food taste differently from pan-fried or deep-fried food?

Ideally, there should be no noticeable difference in texture and taste between air-fried food and traditionally fried food. The outer part is brown and crispy while the inside can be soft or tender.

At most, air-fried food should be lighter since less oil has been used to cook it. The differences, however, would be highlighted depending on the cooking technique, such the usage of oil sprayers instead of a brush and the type of breading used to coat the food.

Question #4
Where can I buy an air fryer?

Due to its growing popularity in recent years, you can now purchase an air fryer from any major appliance store. There are dozens of brands and hundreds of models to choose from, so you should do careful research on the reviews from customers who already own the said air fryer. Take note of the special features, available accessories, and service warranty for each model that you are interested in.

There are also online shops that offer air fryers, but you have to be careful if you decide to go this way. Some offer relatively cheap models from unknown brands. Similarly, you should carefully evaluate a second-hand air fryer, and check for any existing issues or damages. Opting to save money instead of going for quality can cause you headaches later on, and in some cases, may even be a fire hazard in your home.

Question #5

Do I need accessories to cook or bake using the air fryer?

It is not required, but making use of certain accessories can improve the results or quicken the cooking time. Before even buying such accessories, check first if they are compatible with a particular model of the air fryer. Typically, the manufacturer offers accessories that may only be used for the brands that they carry. Common examples of the air fryer accessories include a grill mat, which can keep the basket free from charred food particles, and the baking dish, which is mainly used to cook saucy dishes.

Mistakes to Avoid When Using the Air Fryer

Operating an air fryer does not require much skill. However, you do need to know at least the basics on how to use this in cooking or reheating food properly. Some people just want to dive in and try this out immediately, but such enthusiasm can lead to ruined dinner or, worse, a broken air fryer. You cannot just turn on the machine and expect it to do its thing. There are certain tips and tricks on how you could achieve the perfectly cooked and healthier meal that you are expecting.

Knowing what to avoid is one thing, but you must also learn how to correct these bad practices for the success of your next run. There are cases too that would still allow you to salvage the food that you have been trying to cook. To guide you through this, here is a list of the common mistakes that first-timers make, and how you can avoid or correct them:

Mistake #1

Blocking off the vents for hot air and steam

Any equipment that produces and releases heat needs adequate space for ventilation. It is perfectly alright to store an air fryer in a cabinet, or to place a cover over the top while you are not using it. However, during the cooking process, you must always observe the recommended clearance space of about five inches away from the wall or other objects for all sides.

By giving it room to suck in and vent air, the air fryer would be able to function better and faster. It would also prevent the occurrence of fire due to overheating.

Mistake #2

Not preheating the air fryer before cooking the food

Unlike microwave ovens, air fryer cannot be used right away to cook, bake, or reheat food. Skipping the preheating process would always result to a greasy and soggy mess that you would not want to eat.

According to experts, preheating the air fryer for at least ten minutes before putting in the food is enough to get the perfect color and crisp that you want to achieve. By letting the air fryer achieve a certain temperature first, the heat inside would make the cooking process more effective and efficient. This means that the outer surface would become golden brown and crispy, while the inside is cooked well and tender.

Mistake #3
Using Traditional Types of Batter

There are certain recipes that call for a wet and loose batter, such as corndogs and churros. Cooking such dishes is best done through either pan frying or deep frying. Attempting to do so with an air fryer would be a disaster since the batter would drip down or get blown by the hot air to the bottom of the basket.

The best types of coating for air-fried food are those made of breadcrumbs or dough. Many suggest following the three-step breading procedure:

- Coat the food with flour and seasoning.
- Dip flour-coated food into a whole beaten egg.
- Coat food with breadcrumbs.

You should spray oil onto your breaded food to ensure its crispiness and golden brown appearance. Avoid using the same amount of oil that you normally use for regular frying since this would end up ruining the quality of the food instead.

Mistake #4
Applying dry seasoning to the food

Due to the technology used for air fryers, using dry seasoning to flavor your food is not advisable. The hot air circulating inside the air fryer would only blow away the seasoning, which would result to bland food and a dirty air fryer basket.

To prevent this, make sure that there is something to adhere the seasoning to the surface of the food. For example, you can sprinkle salt and pepper on your vegetables after you have given them a spray or two of cooking oil. For breaded dishes, dip each piece into beaten eggs before frying.

Mistake #5
Using the air fryer to cook fresh vegetables

Most people buy an air fryer to make their meals healthier while still retaining the delicious texture and taste of fried food. Many beginners, however, are disappointed when their attempts to cook fresh vegetables using the air fryer result to charred, dry meals instead.

If you want fried vegetables cooked with your air fryer, then go for the frozen variants instead of fresh ones. The extra moisture inside the frozen vegetables turn into steam during the cooking process, ensuring that the food is cooked all the way through. Do not be afraid of using frozen vegetables since they still have almost the same quality and nutrients as those contained by their fresh counterparts.

Mistake #6
Putting too many items in the basket at one time

Much like a regular frying pan, it is not a good idea to overcrowd the basket of an air fryer. If there are too many pieces being fried at the same time, the results would be uneven—half would likely be burnt, while the rest would end up undercooked.

To correct this practice, try putting your food into manageable batches. For an air fryer, you should not fill up more than half the basket in one go. If you need to cook a large amount of food—in case you're having a dinner party or if you have a huge family to feed—it is best to plan ahead the schedule of your preparation and cooking time. Keep in mind as well that larger models of air fryers mean that you can cook more per batch.

Mistake #7
Not using oil at all, or not using enough oil

One of the primary selling points of an air fryer is its promise of oil-free cooking. Technically, yes, you may cook food in it without using oil. However, the outcome will not be what you are probably envisioning—crispy and golden brown. Instead, you will likely end up with soggy and pale, albeit a bit healthier, food.

To achieve the right balance of taste, texture, and quality, use at least a couple teaspoons of vegetable oil or any other high quality oil. If you are keen on cooking without oil, then you may try using a non-stick cooking spray instead.

You must brush or spray oil onto the food items that you would be cooking before arranging them in the basket. This would keep the interiors of the air fryer relatively clean and free from excessive grease.

Mistake #8
Using too much oil

Though you have to use oil to achieve the best results using an air fryer, you should be careful not to overdo it. If you do not use spray or brush to apply oil, you might end up using the same amount of cooking oil that you typically use for traditional means of frying.

Unlike regular frying, adding more oil will not result to crispiness. Instead, you are likely going to get a burnt, greasy mess. Do not give in to the temptation of adding more oil to improve the quality of the food you are cooking. One or two teaspoons would do, most of the time. If you are still not getting the quality that you are expecting, then this might be due to another air fryer issue.

Mistake #9
Not using the air fryer accessories

Most recipes only require you to arrange the food onto the air fryer basket. However, to get the most out of your fryers, consider using the accessories available for the model you have purchased.

For example, to get better results when you use the air fryer for baking, there are baking accessories that are designed specially to fit inside the air fryer basket. In relation to that, making muffins using the air fryer is best done by using a silicon mold for each.

There are also accessories that can make the cleaning process more efficient. Wax paper liners and oil sprayers are used to prevent food particles from sticking to the sides and bottom of the basket.

Mistake #10

Forgetting to flip the food halfway through the cooking or baking time

Many buy an air fryer since it is being marketed as the healthier and more convenient way of frying food. This is accurate, but it does not mean that you can just throw in the food at the start and get the perfect meal without further effort on your part.

If you are following a recipe, follow the directions carefully since almost every recipe requires for the food to be flipped over at a certain point. This would ensure that both sides would be browned well and turn crispy outside while staying tender inside.

You may pull out the air fryer basket in the middle of cooking to check the status of your food. You can even spray a bit more oil if the color of the food is not up to your expectation. Just be careful not to burn yourself with the hot surface of the air fryer and the even hotter steam that would emanate from the basket.

Mistake #11

Not using the air fryer to bake breads and pastries

The name itself might cause new users to overlook the other functionalities of an air fryer. However, if you have done your research carefully, then you would certainly come across recipes for breads and pastries that are baked using the air fryer. This is made possible since the technology used for air fryer is similar to the one used for conventional ovens.

To use an air fryer for baking, simply follow the recipe that you have found, even the prescribed baking time. The main limiting factor for this, however, is the size of the air fryer basket that you have. Since this equipment is designed to be portable, the space available is smaller compared to traditional ovens.

Experienced users use silicon molds and ramekins to made individual-sized portions. If not, they divide their dough or mixtures into smaller batches and then bake them accordingly. If there is no mold or container to hold the item inside the air fryer, you must use a pan or liner to prevent the food from being melted through the holes of the basket.

Mistake #12

Not cleaning it properly after each use

Since the air fryer does not leave as much oil and grease as a regular frying pan after each use, you might begin to think that it is perfectly alright to leave it in that state. Worse, you might even believe that it is okay to use it again without cleaning it first.

By leaving the grease and crumbs inside the air fryer, you are running the risk of burning the next food item that you would cook in it. Also, as the leftover food particles become charred, they would begin to emit dark and smelly streams of smoke. You would end up ruining both your meal and the ambiance of your kitchen.

Rather than storing away the air fryer right after each use, you must wash each part of it using warm water and dishwashing liquid. The air fryer cannot be washed and dried through a machine, so you have to hand wash every part and wipe everything dry using a clean towel.

To keep you from making these mistakes, always read the manual first before attempting to use the air fryer. If you are not sure if a recipe or method would work, refer to the various air frying blogs and articles found in the Internet. It is best to leave out the experiments to experienced users for now so that you would not waste food or even damage your air fryer. Once you get the hang of it, you are free to try out new techniques and recipes to get the most out of your air fryer.

Measurement Conversion Table

Measurement	Conversion
1 stick of butter	1/2 cup or 8 tablespoons
4 quarts	1 gallon
2 quarts	1/2 gallon
1 cup	8 fluid ounces or 1/2 pint or 16 tablespoons
2 cups	1 pint
1 quart	32 ounces or 2 pints or 4 cups
4 tablespoons	1/4 cup
8 tablespoons	1/2 cup
1/2 tablespoon	1 1/2 teaspoons
3 teaspoons	1 tablespoon

Breakfast Recipes

"The Bomb" Breakfast Balls

Nutritional Facts: *Calories 305 Fat 15.0 g Protein 19.0 g Carbohydrates 26.0 g*

Prep time: 20 min **Cook time**: *25 min*

Servings: 2

Ingredients:

- Pizza dough, whole wheat, freshly prepared (4 ounces)
- Eggs, large, lightly beaten (3 pieces)
- Chives, fresh, chopped (1 tablespoon)
- Bacon slices, center cut (3 pieces)
- Cream cheese, 1/3-reduced-fat, softened (1 ounce)
- Cooking spray

Directions:

1. Cook the bacon over medium heat until crisp and browned. Crumble and set aside in a bowl.
2. Cook eggs in the bacon fat until almost set. Add eggs to the bowl filled with crumbled bacon. Stir along with the chives and cream cheese.
3. Cut pizza dough into four pieces, then roll to form 5-inch rounds. Fill each dough round with egg mixture (1/4 portion). Brush water on the edges before wrapping and pinching into a purse.
4. Add dough purses into the air fryer to cook for five minutes at 350 degrees Fahrenheit.

Scrumptious Sweet Potato Hash

Nutritional Facts: *Calories 191 Fat 6.0 g Protein 3.7 g Carbohydrates 31.4 g*

Prep Time: 10 min **Cook time:** *15 min*

Servings: 6

Ingredients:

- Paprika, smoked (1 tablespoon)
- Bacon slices, chopped into tiny bits (2 pieces)
- Black pepper, freshly ground (1 teaspoon)
- Sweet potato, large, sliced into one-inch cubes (2 pieces)
- Olive oil, extra virgin (2 tablespoons)
- Sea salt (1 teaspoon)
- Dill weed, dried (1 teaspoon)

Directions:

1. Set the air fryer at 400 degrees Fahrenheit to preheat.
2. Combine the sweet potato with bacon, pepper, salt, olive oil, dill, and paprika.
3. Add the sweet potato mixture to the air fryer and cook for twelve to sixteen minutes.

Easy Hash Browns

Nutritional Facts: *Calories 186 Fat 4.3 g Protein 4.0 g Carbohydrates 33.70 g*

Prep Time: *15 min* **Cook time:** *30 min*

Servings: *4*

Ingredients:

- Olive oil, extra virgin (1 tablespoon)
- Seasoning mix, taco (1/2 teaspoon)
- Jalapeno, w/ seeds removed, sliced into one-inch rings (1 piece)
- Salt (1/4 teaspoon)
- Black pepper, freshly ground (1/4 teaspoon)
- Potatoes, peeled, sliced into one-inch chunks (1 ½ pounds)
- Onion, small, sliced into one-inch chunks (1 piece)
- Olive oil, extra virgin (1/2 teaspoon)
- Cumin, ground (1/2 teaspoon)
- Bell pepper, red, w/ seeds removed, sliced into one-inch portions (1 piece)

Directions:

1. Let the potatoes sit in cold water for twenty minutes. Meanwhile, set the air fryer at 320 degrees Fahrenheit to preheat.
2. Drain, pat dry, and coat the potatoes with olive oil (1 tablespoon). Cook in the air fryer for eighteen minutes.
3. Toss the onion, jalapeno pepper, and bell pepper with olive oil (1/2 teaspoon), ground cumin, pepper, salt, and taco seasoning.
4. Combine the air-fried potatoes with the veggie mixture. Place in the air fryer and cook this time at 365 degrees Fahrenheit for ten minutes.

Doughnuts-To-Go

Nutritional Facts: *Calories 238 Fat 4.0 g Protein 5.0 g Carbohydrates 46.0 g*

Prep Time: *45 min* **Cook time:** *35 min*

Servings: *8*

Ingredients:

- Tap water (4 teaspoons)
- Dry yeast, active (1 teaspoon)
- Sugar, powdered (1 cup)
- Milk, whole, at room temp. (1/4 cup)
- Flour, all purpose (2 cups)
- Egg, large, beaten (1 piece)
- Water, warmed to 100 to 100 degrees Fahrenheit (1/4 cup)
- Sugar, granulated, divided (1/4 cup + ½ teaspoon)
- Salt, kosher (1/4 teaspoon)
- Butter, unsalted, melted (2 tablespoons)

Directions:

1. Mix the yeast and granulated sugar (1/2 teaspoon) with water. Let stand to foam up.
2. Mix the remaining granulated sugar (1/4 cup) with salt and flour. Stir in the butter, egg, milk, and prepared yeast mixture to form a soft dough.

3. Knead the dough on a floured surface. Once smooth, place in a covered bowl and set aside to rise and double in size.
4. Roll the dough out until it is a quarter-of-an-inch-thick. Use a 3-inch circle cutter to make 8 rounds, then use a 1-inch circle cutter to cut out their centers. Let the 8 doughnuts and 8 doughnut holes rise, covered loosely, for half an hour on a floured surface.
5. Working in batches, cook the doughnut pieces in the air fryer for four to five minutes at 350 degrees Fahrenheit.
6. Whisk tap water and powdered sugar together to form a smooth glaze. Dip the doughnut pieces in the glaze, then let stand to allow the glaze to harden.
7. Serve and enjoy.

Breakfast Cheese Rolls

Nutritional Facts: Calories 97 Fat 5.5 g Protein 2.7 g Carbohydrates 9.2 g

Prep Time: 15 min **Cook time:** 10 min

Servings: 20

Ingredients:

- Manioc starch (3/4 cup)
- Salt (1 teaspoon)
- Water (1/4 cup)
- Cheddar cheese, shredded (3/4 cup)
- Manioc starch, sweet (3/4 cup)
- Milk, whole (1 /4 cup)
- Olive oil, extra virgin (1/4 cup)
- Eggs, beaten lightly (2 pieces)
- Parmigiano-Reggiano cheese, grated finely (1/2 cup)

Directions:

1. Set the air fryer at 325 degrees Fahrenheit to preheat.
2. Combine the sour manioc and sweet manioc starches.
3. Combine milk with salt, olive oil, and water, then heat until boiling. Lower heat before stirring in the starches. Keep stirring until you have an extremely dry mixture. Let cool.
4. Stir the eggs into the cooled starch mixture to form a smooth dough. Mix well with the Parmigiano-Reggiano and Cheddar cheeses before shaping into golf-ball-sized pieces.
5. Cook dough pieces in the parchment-lined air fryer for eight to ten minutes.

Bananarama Breakfast Bread

Nutritional Facts: Calories 180 Fat 6.0 g Protein 4.0 g Carbohydrates 29.0 g

Prep Time: 20 min **Cook time:** 15 min

Servings: 8

Ingredients:

- Cinnamon (1 teaspoon)
- Eggs, large, beaten lightly (2 pieces)

- Vanilla extract (1 teaspoon)
- Baking soda (1/4 teaspoon)
- Yogurt, nonfat, plain (1/3 cup)
- Walnuts, toasted, chopped coarsely (2 tablespoons)
- Flour, whole wheat, white (3/4 cup)
- Salt, kosher (1/2 teaspoon)
- Bananas, medium, ripe, mashed (2 pieces)
- Sugar, granulated (1/2 cup)
- Vegetable oil (2 tablespoons)
- Cooking spray

Directions:

1. Set the air fryer at 310 degrees Fahrenheit to preheat.
2. Mix the flour with baking soda, cinnamon, and salt.
3. Whisk the eggs together with the mashed bananas, yogurt, sugar, vanilla, and oil. Stir in the flour mixture to form your smooth batter.
4. Pour batter into a parchment-lined round cake pan (6-inch). Top with the walnuts and air-fry for thirty to thirty-five minutes.
5. Let cool before slicing. Serve right away.

Heartwarming Breakfast Buns

Nutritional Facts: *Calories 230 Fat 0.5 g Protein 10.5 g Carbohydrates 46.0 g*

Prep Time: *35 min* **Cook time:** *25 min*

Servings: *4*

Ingredients:

- Baking powder (2 teaspoons)
- Greek yogurt, nonfat, plain (1 cup)
- Cinnamon (3/4 teaspoon)
- Egg white/whole egg, beaten (1 piece)
- Flour, all purpose, unbleached, whole wheat/gluten free (1 cup)
- Raw sugar (2 tablespoons)
- Kosher salt (1/2 teaspoon)
- Raisins (3 tablespoons)

Icing (reserve half):

- Water/milk (1 teaspoon)
- Powdered sugar (1/4 cup)

Directions:

1. Prepare the icing by whisking together the milk and powdered sugar. Pour the smooth mixture into a Ziploc bag.
2. Set the air fryer at 325 degrees Fahrenheit to preheat.
3. Cook the iced rolls in the air fryer for eleven to twelve minutes. Let cool.
4. Trim off the tip of the icing bag. Pipe the icing onto the rolls' surfaces in your desired pattern. (Reserve the remaining icing for another recipe.)

Breakfast Bagels

Nutritional Facts: Calories 152 Fat 0.3 g Protein 10.0 g Carbohydrates 26.5 g

Prep Time: 5 min **Cook time:** 25 min

Servings: 4

Ingredients:

- Baking powder (2 teaspoons)
- Flour, all purpose, whole wheat/gluten free, unbleached (1 cup)
- Greek yogurt, nonfat (1 cup)
- Kosher salt (3/4 teaspoon)
- Egg white, beaten (1 piece)

Toppings:

- Sesame seeds
- Dried garlic flakes
- Poppy seeds
- Dried onion flakes
- Other bagel seasonings

Directions:

1. Set the air fryer at 280 degrees Fahrenheit to preheat.
2. Whisk the flour, salt, and baking powder well. Stir in the yogurt to form a crumbly dough.
3. Turn out the dough onto a floured surface and knead until tacky. Shape into 4 balls, then roll each ball to form ¾-inch-thick cylinders that you join at the ends to make your bagels.
4. Brush bagels with egg wash before sprinkling with desired topping (not included in this recipe's calorie count). Place in the preheated air fryer and cook for fifteen minutes.

Filling Frittata

Nutritional Facts: Calories 233 Fat 15.0 g Protein 17.0 g Carbohydrates 6.0 g

Prep Time: 10 min **Cook time:** 15 min

Servings: 2

Ingredients:

- Milk (1/2 cup)
- Black pepper, freshly ground (1/2 teaspoon)
- Bell pepper, red, chopped (1/4 cup)
- Mushrooms, baby bella, chopped (1/4 cup)
- Salt (1/2 teaspoon)
- Eggs (4 pieces)
- Green onions, chopped (2 pieces)
- Spinach, chopped (1/4 cup)
- Cheddar cheese (1/4 cup)
- Hot sauce (1/4 teaspoon)

Directions:

1. Blend the milk and eggs by whisking well. Stir in the black pepper, salt, red bell pepper, hot sauce, green onions, cheddar cheese, spinach, and mushrooms.
2. Pour the egg mixture into a greased round pan (6x3-inch).

3. Cook in the air fryer for fifteen to eighteen minutes at 360 degrees Fahrenheit.

Biscuit Bombs

Nutritional Facts: Calories 190 Fat 13.0 g Protein 7.0 g Carbohydrates 13.0 g

Prep Time: 30 min *Cook time:* 15 min

Servings: 10

Ingredients:

- Salt (1/8 teaspoon)
- Breakfast sausage, bulk (1/4 pound)
- Refrigerated biscuits, canned, flaky (10 1/5 ounces)
- Vegetable oil (1 tablespoon)

- Eggs, beaten (2 pieces)
- Pepper (1/8 teaspoon)
- Cheddar cheese, sharp, sliced into half-inch cubes (2 ounces)

Egg wash:

- Water (1 tablespoon)
- Egg (1 piece)

Directions:

1. Line the air fryer basket with parchment before coating with cooking spray.
2. Cook the sausage in oil until browned and crumbly. Set aside in a bowl.
3. In the same pan, stir the beaten eggs, pepper, and salt together and cook until moist and thickened. Add to the sausage bowl and mix well.
4. Separate the dough and press into 10 four-inch rounds. Fill each round with the egg mixture (1 tablespoon), then add a piece of cheese on top. Fold and pinch to seal before brushing with egg wash.
5. Add 5 biscuit bombs to the air fryer basket. Cover with another parchment paper coated with cooking spray, then place the remaining 5 biscuit bombs on top. Cook for eight minutes.
6. Remove the top parchment paper and arrange all biscuit bombs in a single layer. Air-fry for another four to six minutes.

Lunch Recipes

Yogurt Garlic Chicken

Nutritional Facts: Calories 380 Fat 15.0 g Protein 26.0 g Carbohydrates 34.0 g

Prep Time: 30 min *Cook time:* 60 min

Servings: 6

Ingredients:

- Pita bread rounds, halved (6 pieces)
- English cucumber, sliced thinly, w/ each slice halved (1 cup)

Chicken & vegetables:

- Olive oil (3 tablespoons)
- Black pepper, freshly ground (1/2 teaspoon)
- Chicken thighs, skinless, boneless (20 ounces)
- Bell pepper, red, sliced into half-inch portions (1 piece)
- Garlic cloves, chopped finely (4 pieces)
- Cumin, ground (1/2 teaspoon)
- Red onion, medium, sliced into half-inch wedges (1 piece)
- Yogurt, plain, fat free (1/2 cup)
- Lemon juice (2 tablespoons)
- Salt (1 ½ teaspoons)
- Red pepper flakes, crushed (1/2 teaspoon)
- Allspice, ground (1/2 teaspoon)
- Bell pepper, yellow, sliced into half-inch portions (1 piece)

Yogurt sauce:

- Olive oil (2 tablespoons)
- Salt (1/4 teaspoon)
- Parsley, flat leaf, chopped finely (1 tablespoon)
- Yogurt, plain, fat free (1 cup)
- Lemon juice, fresh (1 tablespoon)
- Garlic clove, chopped finely (1 piece)

Directions:

- Mix the yogurt (1/2 cup), garlic cloves (4 pieces), olive oil (1 tablespoon), salt (1 teaspoon), lemon juice (2 tablespoons), pepper (1/4 teaspoon), allspice, cumin, and pepper flakes. Stir in the chicken and coat well. Cover and marinate in the fridge for two hours.
- Preheat the air fryer at 400 degrees Fahrenheit.
- Grease a rimmed baking sheet (18x13-inch) with cooking spray.
- Toss the bell peppers and onion with remaining olive oil (2 tablespoons), pepper (1/4 teaspoon), and salt (1/2 teaspoon).
- Arrange veggies on the baking sheet's left side and the marinated chicken thighs (drain first) on the right side. Cook in the air fryer for twenty-five to thirty minutes.
- Mix the yogurt sauce ingredients.
- Slice air-fried chicken into half-inch strips.
- Top each pita round with chicken strips, roasted veggies, cucumbers, and yogurt sauce.

Lemony Parmesan Salmon

Nutritional Facts: Calories 290 Fat 16.0 g Protein 33.0 g Carbohydrates 4.0 g

Prep Time: 10 min **Cook time:** 25 min

Servings: 4

Ingredients:

- Butter, melted (2 tablespoons)
- Green onions, sliced thinly (2 tablespoons)
- Breadcrumbs, white, fresh (3/4 cup)
- Thyme leaves, dried (1/4 teaspoon)
- Salmon fillet, 1 ¼-pound (1 piece)
- Salt (1/4 teaspoon)
- Parmesan cheese, grated (1/4 cup)
- Lemon peel, grated (2 teaspoons)

Directions:

- Preheat the air fryer at 350 degrees Fahrenheit.
- Mist cooking spray onto a baking pan (shallow). Fill with pat-dried salmon. Brush salmon with butter (1 tablespoon) before sprinkling with salt.
- Combine the breadcrumbs with onions, thyme, lemon peel, cheese, and remaining butter (1 tablespoon).
- Cover salmon with the breadcrumb mixture. Air-fry for fifteen to twenty-five minutes.

Easiest Tuna Cobbler Ever

Nutritional Facts: Calories 320 Fat 11.0 g Protein 28.0 g Carbohydrates 31.0 g

Prep Time: 15 min **Cook time:** 25 min

Servings: 4

Ingredients:

- Water, cold (1/3 cup)
- Tuna, canned, drained (10 ounces)
- Sweet pickle relish (2 tablespoons)
- Mixed vegetables, frozen (1 ½ cups)
- Soup, cream of chicken, condensed (10 ¾ ounces)
- Pimientos, sliced, drained (2 ounces)
- Lemon juice (1 teaspoon)
- Paprika

Directions:

- Preheat the air fryer at 375 degrees Fahrenheit.
- Mist cooking spray into a round casserole (1 ½ quarts).
- Mix the frozen vegetables with milk, soup, lemon juice, relish, pimientos, and tuna in a saucepan. Cook for six to eight minutes over medium heat.

- Fill the casserole with the tuna mixture.
- Mix the biscuit mix with cold water to form a soft dough. Beat for half a minute before dropping by four spoonfuls into the casserole.
- Dust the dish with paprika before air-frying for twenty to twenty-five minutes.

Deliciously Homemade Pork Buns

Nutritional Facts: Calories 240 Fat 9.0 g Protein 8.0 g Carbohydrates 29.0 g

Prep Time: 20 min *Cook time:* 25 min

Servings: 8

Ingredients:

- Green onions, sliced thinly (3 pieces)
- Egg, beaten (1 piece)
- Pulled pork, diced, w/ barbecue sauce (1 cup)
- Buttermilk biscuits, refrigerated (16 1/3 ounces)
- Soy sauce (1 teaspoon)

Directions:

- Preheat the air fryer at 325 degrees Fahrenheit.
- Use parchment paper to line your baking sheet.
- Combine pork with green onions.
- Separate and press the dough to form 8 four-inch rounds.
- Fill each biscuit round's center with two tablespoons of pork mixture. Cover with the dough edges and seal by pinching. Arrange the buns on the sheet and brush with a mixture of soy sauce and egg.
- Cook in the air fryer for twenty to twenty-five minutes.

Mouthwatering Tuna Melts

Nutritional Facts: Calories 320 Fat 18.0 g Protein 14.0 g Carbohydrates 27.0 g

Prep Time: 15 min *Cook time:* 20 min

Servings: 8

Ingredients:

- Salt (1/8 teaspoon)
- Onion, chopped (1/3 cup)
- Biscuits, refrigerated, flaky layers (16 1/3 ounces)
- Tuna, water packed, drained (10 ounces)
- Mayonnaise (1/3 cup)
- Pepper (1/8 teaspoon)
- Cheddar cheese, shredded (4 ounces)
- Tomato, chopped
- Sour cream
- Lettuce, shredded

Directions:

- Preheat the air fryer at 325 degrees Fahrenheit.
- Mist cooking spray onto a cookie sheet.
- Mix tuna with mayonnaise, pepper, salt, and onion.
- Separate dough so you have 8 biscuits; press each into 5-inch rounds.
- Arrange 4 biscuit rounds on the sheet. Fill at the center with tuna mixture before topping with cheese. Cover with the remaining biscuit rounds and press to seal.
- Air-fry for fifteen to twenty minutes. Slice each sandwich into halves. Serve each piece topped with lettuce, tomato, and sour cream.

Bacon Wings

Nutritional Facts: Calories 100 Fat 5.0 g Protein 10.0 g Carbohydrates 2.0 g

Prep Time: 15 min **Cook time:** 1 hr 15 min

Servings: 12

Ingredients:

- Bacon strips (12 pieces)
- Paprika (1 teaspoon)
- Black pepper (1 tablespoon)
- Oregano (1 teaspoon)
- Chicken wings (12 pieces)
- Kosher salt (1 tablespoon)
- Brown sugar (1 tablespoon)
- Chili powder (1 teaspoon)
- Celery sticks
- Blue cheese dressing

Directions:

- Preheat the air fryer at 325 degrees Fahrenheit.
- Mix sugar, salt, chili powder, oregano, pepper, and paprika. Coat chicken wings with this dry rub.
- Wrap a bacon strip around each wing. Arrange wrapped wings in the air fryer basket.
- Cook for thirty minutes on each side in the air fryer. Let cool for five minutes.
- Serve and enjoy with celery and blue cheese.

Pepper Pesto Lamb

Nutritional Facts: Calories 310 Fat 15.0 g Protein 40.0 g Carbohydrates 1.0 g

Prep Time: 15 min **Cook time:** 1 hr 15 min

Servings: 12

Ingredients:

Pesto:

- Rosemary leaves, fresh (1/4 cup)
- Garlic cloves (3 pieces)
- Parsley, fresh, packed firmly (3/4 cup)
- Mint leaves, fresh (1/4 cup)
- Olive oil (2 tablespoons)

Lamb:

- Red bell peppers, roasted, drained (7 ½ ounces)
- Leg of lamb, boneless, rolled (5 pounds)
- Seasoning, lemon pepper (2 teaspoons)

Directions:

- Preheat the oven at 325 degrees Fahrenheit.
- Mix the pesto ingredients in the food processor.
- Unroll the lamb and cover the cut side with pesto. Top with roasted peppers before rolling up the lamb and tying with kitchen twine.
- Coat lamb with seasoning (lemon pepper) and air-fry for one hour.

Tuna Spinach Casserole

Nutritional Facts: Calories 400 Fat 19.0 g Protein 21.0 g Carbohydrates 35.0 g

Prep Time: 30 min **Cook time:** 25 min

Servings: 8

Ingredients:

- Mushroom soup, creamy (18 ounces)
- Milk (1/2 cup)
- White tuna, solid, in-water, drained (12 ounces)
- Crescent dinner rolls, refrigerated (8 ounces)
- Egg noodles, wide, uncooked (8 ounces)
- Cheddar cheese, shredded (8 ounces)
- Spinach, chopped, frozen, thawed, drained (9 ounces)
- Lemon peel grated (2 teaspoons)

Directions:

- Preheat the oven at 350 degrees Fahrenheit.
- Mist cooking spray onto a glass baking dish (11x7-inch).
- Follow package directions in cooking and draining the noodles.
- Stir the cheese (1 ½ cups) and soup together in a skillet heated on medium. Once cheese melts, stir in your noodles, milk, spinach, tuna, and lemon peel. Once bubbling, pour into the prepped dish.
- Unroll the dough and sprinkle with remaining cheese (1/2 cup). Roll up dough and pinch at the seams to seal. Slice into 8 portions and place over the tuna mixture.
- Air-fry for twenty to twenty-five minutes.

Greek Style Mini Burger Pies

Nutritional Facts: Calories 270 Fat 15.0 g Protein 19.0 g Carbohydrates 13.0 g

Prep Time: 15 min **Cook time:** 40 min

Servings: 6

Ingredients:

Burger mixture:

- Onion, large, chopped (1 piece)
- Red bell peppers, roasted, diced (1/2 cup)

- Ground lamb, 80% lean (1 pound)
- Red pepper flakes (1/4 teaspoon)
- Feta cheese, crumbled (2 ounces)

Baking mixture:

- Milk (1/2 cup)
- Biscuit mix, classic (1/2 cup)

- Eggs (2 pieces)

Directions:

- Preheat the air fryer at 350 degrees Fahrenheit.
- Grease 12 muffin cups using cooking spray.
- Cook the onion and beef in a skillet heated on medium-high. Once beef is browned and cooked through, drain and let cool for five minutes. Stir together with feta cheese, roasted red peppers, and red pepper flakes.
- Whisk the baking mixture ingredients together. Fill each muffin cup with baking mixture (1 tablespoon).
- Air-fry for twenty-five to thirty minutes. Let cool before serving.

Family Fun Pizza

Nutritional Facts: Calories 215 Fat 10.0 g Protein 13.0 g Carbohydrates 20.0 g

Prep Time: 30 min *Cook time:* 25 min

Servings: 16

Ingredients:

Pizza crust:

- Water, warm (1 cup)
- Salt (1/2 teaspoon)
- Flour, whole wheat (1 cup)
- Olive oil (2 tablespoons)

- Dry yeast, quick active (1 package)
- Flour, all purpose (1 ½ cups)
- Cornmeal
- Olive oil

Filling:

- Onion, chopped (1 cup)
- Mushrooms, sliced, drained (4 ounces)
- Garlic cloves, chopped finely (2 pieces)
- Parmesan cheese, grated (1/4 cup)

- Ground lamb, 80% lean (1 pound)
- Italian seasoning (1 teaspoon)
- Pizza sauce (8 ounces)
- Mozzarella cheese, shredded (2 cups)

Directions:

- Mix yeast with warm water. Combine with flours, oil (2 tablespoons), and salt by stirring and then beating vigorously for half a minute. Let the dough sit for twenty minutes.
- Preheat the air fryer at 350 degrees Fahrenheit.
- Prep 2 square pans (8-inch) by greasing with oil before sprinkling with cornmeal.
- Cut the rested dough in half; place each half inside each pan. Set aside, covered, for thirty to forty-five minutes. Cook in the air fryer for twenty to twenty-two minutes.
- Sauté the onion, beef, garlic, and Italian seasoning until beef is completely cooked. Drain and set aside.
- Cover the air-fried crusts with pizza sauce before topping with beef mixture, cheeses, and mushrooms.
- Return to the air fryer and cook for twenty minutes.

Air Fryer Accessory #1

If you own a Philips Airfryer, Power AirFryer, Farberware airfryer or other airfryers, the below collection offers a unique selection of accessories perfectly curated to complement your cooking!

This collection consists of:

Cake Barrel

Pizza Pan

Silicone Egg Bites Mould

Double Layer Rack

Barbecue Rack

Toast Rack

For more information about this collection go to:

www.MillenniumPublishingLimited.com > Barbara Trisler > Air Fryer Accessories

Dinner Recipes

Crispy Italian Style Chicken with Tomato Arugula Salad

Nutritional Facts: Calories 390 Fat 17.0 g Protein 36.0 g Carbohydrates 22.0 g

Prep Time: 20 min **Cook time:** 30 min

Servings: 4

Ingredients:

- Egg (1 piece)
- Parmesan cheese, grated (1/4 cup)
- Salt (1/4 teaspoon)
- Basil leaves, fresh, sliced thinly (2 tablespoons)
- Flour, all purpose (2 tablespoons)
- Balsamic vinegar (1 tablespoon)
- Breadcrumbs, crispy, Italian style panko (3/4 cup)
- Chicken thighs, skinless, boneless (20 ounces)

Tomato arugula salad:

- Balsamic vinegar (1 teaspoon)
- Pepper (1/8 teaspoon)
- Cherry tomatoes, halved (1 cup)
- Olive, extra virgin (2 tablespoons)
- Salt (1/4 teaspoon)
- Baby arugula (4 cups)

Directions:

- Line air fryer basket with parchment. Preheat at 300 degrees Fahrenheit.
- Fill a shallow dish with flour; another dish with a beaten mixture of egg, salt (1/4 teaspoon), and vinegar (1 tablespoon); and another dish with a mixture of Parmesan and breadcrumbs.
- Dip chicken in flour before coating with egg mixture and covering with breadcrumb mixture.
- Cook chicken in air fryer for fifteen minutes on each side.
- Combine vinegar (1 teaspoon), salt (1/4 teaspoon), pepper, and olive oil in a large bowl. Toss in tomatoes and arugula.
- Serve chicken with salad.

Feta Orzo and Lamb Chops

Nutritional Facts: Calories 390 Fat 13.0 g Protein 33.0 g Carbohydrates 36.0 g

Prep Time: 5 min **Cook time:** 30 min

Servings: 4

Ingredients:

- Lemon juice, fresh (1 tablespoon)
- Garlic cloves, chopped finely (4 pieces)
- Lamb loin chops, ¼-pound, fat-trimmed (8 pieces)

- Salt (1/2 teaspoon)
- Sundried tomatoes, oil-packed, drained, chopped finely (2 tablespoons)
- Orzo/rosamarina pasta, uncooked (1 cup)
- Oregano leaves, dried (1 tablespoon)
- Pepper (1/2 teaspoon)
- Feta cheese, basil-tomato, crumbled (1/3 cup)

Directions:

- Preheat air fryer at 375 degrees Fahrenheit.
- Follow package direction in cooking pasta without adding oil and salt. Drain and keep warm.
- Combine salt (1/4 teaspoon), pepper, garlic, and oregano. Rub mixture all over lamb chops.
- Cook lamb chops in air fryer for 30 minutes, turning halfway.
- Toss pasta with tomatoes, oil, cheese, lemon juice, and remaining pepper (1/4 teaspoon) and salt (1/4 teaspoon). Serve with the lamb chops.

Comforting Tuna Bake

Nutritional Facts: Calories 400 Fat 14.0 g Protein 22.0 g Carbohydrates 45.0 g

Prep Time: 20 min **Cook time:** 35 min

Servings: 6

Ingredients:

- Sweet peas, frozen (1 ½ cups)
- Seasoned salt (1 teaspoon)
- Evaporated milk (12 ounces) OR half-and-half (1 ½ cups)
- Onions, French fried (2 4/5 ounces)
- Egg noodles, wide, uncooked (4 cups)
- Soup, cream of celery, condensed (10 ¾ ounces)
- Onion, dried, minced (1 tablespoon)
- Tuna, water-packed, drained, flaked (10 ounces)

Directions:

- Follow package directions in cooking noodles. Add peas at last minute. Drain and set aside.
- Preheat air fryer at 325 degrees Fahrenheit.
- Combine soup with milk, seasoned salt, and dried onion in an ungreased casserole (2-quart). Add cooked noodles and toss to combine.
- Cover dish and air-fry for thirty minutes.
- Give dish a stir, add French fried onions on top, and return to air fryer to cook for another five minutes.

Tempting Turkey Caprese Dish

Nutritional Facts: Calories 250 Fat 10.0 g Protein 11.0 g Carbohydrates 28.0 g

Prep Time: 10 min **Cook time:** 30 min

Servings: 8

Ingredients:

- Olive oil (1 tablespoon)
- Deli turkey, sliced thinly, diced (1/2 pound)
- Cherry tomatoes, halved (1 cup)
- Refrigerated biscuits (16 3/10 ounces)
- Mozzarella cheese, shredded (1 cup)
- Black pepper, ground (1 /4 teaspoon)
- Basil leaves, fresh, shredded (1/4 cup)

Directions:

- Preheat air fryer at 350 degrees Fahrenheit.
- Mist cooking spray onto a glass baking dish (3-quart). Fill with dough, separated into 8 biscuits.
- Create 2 X-slits half-inch-deep into each biscuit. Air-fry for seventeen to twenty minutes.
- Combine cheese with turkey.
- Let biscuits cool before forming into cups. Brush each with olive oil and then fill with turkey mixture. Dust with pepper and air-fry for eleven to fourteen minutes.
- Serve sprinkled with basil and tomatoes.

Tender Turkey Meatloaf

Nutritional Facts: Calories 250 Fat 10.0 g Protein 26.0 g Carbohydrates 17.0 g

Prep Time: 15 min *Cook time:* 50 min

Servings: 5

Ingredients:

- Sugar, light brown, packed (1 tablespoon)
- Onion, chopped finely (3/4 cup)
- Breadcrumbs, Italian style (1/4 cup)
- Pepper (1/2 teaspoon)
- Ketchup (1/2 cup)
- Garlic cloves, chopped finely (2 pieces)
- Ketchup (1 teaspoon)
- Vegetable oil (2 teaspoons)
- Green bell pepper, chopped finely (1/4 cup)
- Cheddar cheese, sharp, reduced fat, shredded (1/4 cup)
- Italian seasoning (1 ½ teaspoons)
- Salt (1/2 teaspoon)
- Egg, slightly beaten (1 piece)
- Yellow mustard (1 teaspoon)
- Turkey breast, ground (1 ¼ pounds)

Directions:

- Preheat air fryer at 325 degrees Fahrenheit.
- Grease a loaf pan (8x4-inch) with cooking spray.
- Cook garlic, onion, and bell pepper in oil heated on medium-high for three minutes. Set aside.
- Combine onion mixture with cheese, Italian seasoning, salt, pepper, breadcrumbs, egg, and ketchup (1 teaspoon). Add turkey and mix well.
- Fill loaf pan with turkey mixture. Air-fry for thirty-five minutes.

- Mix mustard with brown sugar and ketchup (1/2 cup) and spread all over meatloaf.
- Return meatloaf to air fryer and cook for five minutes. Rest for ten minutes, slice, and serve.

Baked Chicken Orzo

Nutritional Facts: Calories 440 Fat 17.0 g Protein 29.0 g Carbohydrates 43.0 g

Prep Time: 30 min *Cook time:* 45 min

Servings: 6

Ingredients:

- Queso fresco, crumbled (3/4 cup)
- Chicken broth (1/2 cup)
- Red bell pepper, medium, diced (1 piece)
- Vegetable oil (2 tablespoons)
- Butter (2 tablespoons)
- Salt (1 teaspoon)
- Chicken thighs, skinless, boneless (20 ounces)
- Rosamarina/orzo pasta, uncooked (1/2 pound)
- Chili powder (2 teaspoons)
- White onion, diced (1 cup)
- Jalapeno chile, seeded, chopped finely (1 piece)
- Tomatoes, fire roasted, undrained (14 ½ ounces)
- Taco seasoning mix (1 ounce)
- Cilantro leaves, fresh, chopped (2 tablespoons)

Directions:

- Preheat air fryer at 350 degrees Fahrenheit.
- Use cooking spray to grease a glass baking dish (3-quart).
- Cook pasta, drain, and toss with chili powder and broth.
- Melt butter in skillet heated on medium-high. Stir in onion, jalapeno, bell pepper, and salt. Cook until veggies are browned and soft. Stir in tomatoes and cook until mixture thickens. Toss in cooked pasta.
- Fill baking dish with pasta mixture.
- Toss chicken thighs with taco seasoning mix and vegetable oil. Add on top of pasta mixture.
- Cover dish and air-fry for thirty-five minutes. Serve topped with cilantro and queso fresco.

Potato Spinach Loaf

Nutritional Facts: Calories 290 Fat 6.0 g Protein 12.0 g Carbohydrates 47.0 g

Prep Time: 20 min *Cook time:* 50 min

Servings: 6

Ingredients:

Loaf:

- Mushrooms stems & pieces, drained, chopped (4 ounces)
- Hash brown potatoes, frozen, thawed (4 cups)
- Salt (1/2 teaspoon)
- Breadcrumbs, Italian style (1 cup)
- Black pepper, coarsely ground (1/4 teaspoon)
- Eggs, beaten (3 pieces)
- Spinach, cut, frozen, thawed, drained (2 cups)
- Onion, chopped (1/2 cup)
- Nutmeg (1/8 teaspoon)

Sauce:

- Milk (1/3 cup)
- Soup, cream of mushroom, condensed, w/ roasted garlic & herbs (10 ¾ ounces)

Directions:

- Preheat air fryer at 325 degrees Fahrenheit.
- Mist cooking spray onto a loaf pan (8x4-inch).
- Mix all ingredients and press into pan.
- Air-fry for forty-five to fifty minutes. Let cool for five minutes.
- Stir and cook milk and soup together until heated though and thickened.
- Serve loaf sliced and smothered with sauce.

Garlic Herb Lamb

Nutritional Facts: Calories 275 Fat 13.0 g Protein 39.0 g Carbohydrates 1.0 g

Prep Time: 20 min *Cook time:* 50 min

Servings: 8

Ingredients:

- Garlic cloves, slivered (3 pieces)
- Salt (1 ½ teaspoons)
- Pepper (1/2 teaspoon)
- Lamb leg, 5-pound (1 piece)
- Dill weed, dried (3 teaspoons)
- Rosemary leaves, dried, crushed (1 teaspoon)

Directions:

- Preheat air fryer at 375 degrees Fahrenheit.
- Without removing fell from lamb, create 10 small slits and fill with garlic slivers.
- Combine all other ingredients and rub all over the lamb.
- Air-fry lamb for fifty minutes. Tent with foil and rest for twenty minutes.
- Serve and enjoy.

Hearty Seafood Pot Pie

Nutritional Facts: Calories 300 Fat 4.5 g Protein 20.0 g Carbohydrates 41.0 g

Prep Time: 20 min **Cook time:** 35 min

Servings: 4

Ingredients:

- Salt (1/2 teaspoon)
- Bay scallops (1/2 pound)
- Half-and-half, fat free (2/3 cup)
- Cooking spray, butter flavor
- Basil leaves, chopped coarsely (1/4 cup)
- Shrimp, medium, uncooked, peeled, deveined (1/2 pound)
- Pepper, freshly ground (1/2 teaspoon)
- Soup, cream of mushroom, condensed, 98% fat free, reduced sodium (10 ¾ ounces)
- Baby potato blend, gourmet, frozen, thawed (28 ounces)
- Phyllo pastry sheets, 14x18-inch, frozen, thawed (3 pieces)

Directions:

- Preheat air fryer at 350 degrees Fahrenheit.
- Mist cooking spray onto a glass baking dish (2-quart).
- Toss shrimp along with pepper and scallops, then spray with cooking spray. Cook for two minutes on medium-high, then toss gently with a mixture of half-and-half and soup (whisked together), potato blend, salt, and basil.
- Fill baking dish with seafood mixture. Cover with pastry sheets, placed in alternate crosswise/lengthwise pattern, and misted with cooking spray. Air-fry for thirty minutes.

Festive Pork Roast

Nutritional Facts: Calories 380 Fat 20.0 g Protein 38.0 g Carbohydrates 12.0 g

Prep Time: 30 min **Cook time:** 1 hr 40 min

Servings: 12

Ingredients:

- Cherry/grape tomatoes, sliced in half (1/2 cup)
- Corn, frozen (2 cups)
- Pork loin roast, 4-pound, boneless, fat-trimmed, butterflied (1 piece)
- Cumin, ground (1/2 teaspoon)
- Avocado, ripe, pitted, peeled, cubed (1 piece)
- Cilantro, fresh, chopped (2 tablespoons + 1 teaspoon)
- Taco seasoning mix (1 ounce)
- Lime peel, grated (1 ½ teaspoons)
- Taco shells, crushed into half-inch portions (1 ¼ cups)
- Four-cheese blend, Mexican, shredded (1 ½ cups)
- Green onions, chopped (2 tablespoons)
- Garlic salt (1/2 teaspoon)
- Pepper, freshly cracked (1/4 teaspoon)
- Salt (1/4 teaspoon)

- Chicken broth (1/2 cup)
- Lime juice, fresh (1 tablespoon)
- Lime slices

Directions:

- Preheat air fryer a 325 degrees Fahrenheit.
- Combine crushed taco shells with frozen corn, cilantro, onions, and cheese.
- Sprinkle flat-open pork roast with pepper and salt before covering with taco shell mixture (leave ¾-inch border on the edge uncovered).
- Roll up pork like you would a jelly roll and secure with kitchen string. Cover evenly with taco seasoning mix before placing in air fryer basket. Cook for one hour and thirty minutes. Tent pork roll with foil and let sit for ten minutes.
- Mix remaining corn (1 cup) with cumin, garlic salt, and broth in a baking dish. Cook in the air fryer for two to three minutes. Stir in tomatoes, avocado, lime juice, and lime peel. Cook for two minutes.
- Slice pork. Serve garnished with cilantro and lime, alongside avocado-corn salsa.

Poultry Recipes

Supreme Sesame Chicken

Nutritional Facts: Calories 302 Fat 13.0 g Protein 26.0 g Carbohydrates 18.0 g

Prep Time: 20 min **Cook time:** 15 min

Servings: 4

Ingredients:

- Cornstarch, divided (1/3 cup + 2 teaspoons)
- Soy sauce, reduced sodium (2 tablespoons)
- Canola oil (1 ½ tablespoons)
- Chiles de árbol, seeded, chopped (3 pieces)
- White pepper, freshly ground (1/4 teaspoon)
- Sesame seeds, toasted (1/2 teaspoon)
- Sugar (2 teaspoons)
- Green onion, sliced thinly, divided (2 tablespoons)
- Chicken thighs, skinless, boneless, patted dry, sliced into one-inch cubes (1 pound)
- Egg, large (1 piece)
- Salt, kosher (1/4 teaspoon)
- Chicken broth, low-sodium (7 tablespoons)
- Ketchup (2 tablespoons)
- Rice vinegar, unseasoned (2 teaspoons)
- Ginger, fresh, chopped finely (1 tablespoon)
- Garlic, chopped finely (1 tablespoon)
- Sesame oil, toasted (1 teaspoon)

Directions:

- Beat the egg before slathering all over the chicken.

- Mix the cornstarch (1/3 cup) with pepper and salt. Add the egg-coated chicken and stir well.
- Place the chicken in the air fryer (preheated at 400 degrees Fahrenheit) and cook for three to five minutes. Set aside to dry.
- Whisk the remaining cornstarch (2 teaspoons) with sugar, broth, rice vinegar, ketchup, and soy sauce.
- Cook the chiles in canola oil; once sizzling, stir in the garlic and ginger and cook for one minute.
- Stir the cornstarch mixture into the chile mixture. Once the sauce bubbles, stir in the chicken and cook for two minutes. Remove from heat before stirring in the sesame oil and green onion (1 tablespoon).
- Serve sesame chicken topped with remaining green onion (1 tablespoon) and sesame seeds.

Spicy Sweet Chicken Wings

Nutritional Facts: Calories 304 Fat 19.0 g Protein 23.0 g Carbohydrates 8.0 g

Prep Time: 10 min **Cook time:** 20 min

Servings: 2

Ingredients:

- Kosher salt (1/8 teaspoon)
- Chili paste, freshly ground (1 teaspoon)
- Lime juice, freshly squeezed (1 teaspoon)
- Cornstarch (1/2 teaspoon)
- Ginger, fresh, chopped finely (1/2 teaspoon)
- Chicken drumettes (10 pieces)
- Soy sauce, low sodium (1 tablespoon)
- Honey (2 teaspoons)
- Garlic, chopped finely (1 teaspoon)
- Scallions, chopped (2 tablespoons)
- Cooking spray

Directions:

- Pat-dry the chicken before coating with cooking spray.
- Cook in the air fryer for twenty-five minutes at 400 degrees Fahrenheit.
- Whisk the cornstarch and soy sauce together, then whisk in salt, sambal, lime juice, garlic, honey, and ginger. Heat to a simmer until thickened and bubbling.
- Serve chicken coated with the sauce and sprinkled with scallions.

Spiced Up Chicken Thighs

Nutritional Facts: Calories 458 Fat 13.0 g Protein 52.0 g Carbohydrates 36.0 g

Prep Time: 15 min **Cook time:** 35 min

Servings: 4

Ingredients:

- Kosher salt (1/2 teaspoon)
- Paprika (1 teaspoon)
- Eggs, large (2 pieces)
- Hot sauce (2 teaspoons)
- Chicken thighs, skinless, boneless, 6-ounce (4 pieces)
- Panko, whole wheat (2 cups)
- Buttermilk, low fat (2 cups)
- Cayenne pepper (1/2 teaspoon)
- Flour, all purpose (1 cup)
- Water (2 tablespoons)
- Cooking spray

Directions:

- Toss chicken thighs with a mixture of buttermilk, cayenne pepper, and paprika. Marinate in the fridge overnight.
- Fill a shallow dish with flour, a second dish with a mixture of water and whisked eggs, and a third dish with panko.
- Preheat air fryer at 375 degrees Fahrenheit.
- Drain marinated chicken and sprinkle with salt. Coat with flour before dipping in egg mixture and dredging in panko. Mist all chicken pieces with cooking spray.
- Air-fry for sixteen minutes. Serve each chicken piece drizzled with hot sauce (1/2 teaspoon).

Mouthwatering Stuffed Chicken Breast

Nutritional Facts: Calories 185 Fat 8.5 g Protein 14.8 g Carbohydrates 15.2 g

Prep Time: 20 min **Cook time:** 10 min

Servings: 2

Ingredients:

- Jalapeno pepper, fresh, sliced thinly into strips (1 piece)
- Cumin, ground, divided (4 teaspoons)
- Salt (1/4 teaspoon)
- Black pepper, ground (1/4 teaspoon)
- Lime juice (1/2 tablespoon)
- Chipotle flakes (2 teaspoons)
- Onion, sliced thinly into strips (1/2 piece)
- Chili powder, divided (4 teaspoons)
- Chicken breast, boneless, skinless (1 piece)
- Oregano, Mexican (2 teaspoons)
- Bell pepper, red, sliced thinly into strips (1/2 piece)
- Corn oil (2 teaspoons)

Directions:

- Combine cumin (2 teaspoons) and chili powder (2 teaspoons) in a small bowl. Set aside.
- Preheat air fryer at 375 degrees Fahrenheit.
- Gently pound chicken pieces until ¼-inch in thickness. Season with remaining cumin and chili powder, as well as salt, pepper, oregano, and chipotle flakes. Fill each chicken piece with bell pepper (1/2 piece), jalapeno, and onion before rolling and securing with 2 water-soaked toothpicks.
- Coat all roll-ups in the cumin-chili mixture, then drizzle with olive oil. Cook in the air fryer for six minutes on each side.
- Serve drizzled with lime juice.

Crumbed Chicken Tenders with Creamy Basil Sauce

Nutritional Facts (Tenders): Calories 253 Fat 11.4 g Protein 26.2 g Carbohydrates 9.8 g

Nutritional Facts (Sauce): Calories 58 Fat 5.0 g Protein 2.0 g Carbohydrates 2.0 g

Prep Time: 15 min **Cook time:** 12 min

Servings: 4 (1 pc. tender), 1/8 of recipe (1 serving of sauce)

Ingredients:

Tenders:

- Breadcrumbs, dry (1/2 cup)
- Chicken tenderloins (8 pieces)
- Egg (1 piece)
- Vegetable oil (2 tablespoons)

Sauce:

- Salt (1/2 teaspoon)
- Olive oil, extra virgin (1 tablespoon)
- Half-and-half (3/4 cup)
- Garlic clove, medium, chopped finely (1 piece)
- Parmesan cheese, grated finely (2 tablespoons)
- Pepper, ground (1/4 teaspoon)
- Flour, all purpose (1 tablespoon)
- Chicken broth, unsalted (1 cup)
- Basil sprig, fresh, whole (1 piece)
- Basil sprig, fresh, chopped, divided (2 tablespoons)

Directions:

- Preheat air fryer at 325 degrees Fahrenheit.
- Fill a small bowl with whisked egg, and a second bowl with a mixture of oil and breadcrumbs.
- Dip each chicken piece in whisked egg before coating with breadcrumb mixture.
- Air-fry chicken pieces for twelve minutes.
- Stir garlic and flour into oil heated in a saucepan on medium-high. Cook for one minute before adding broth. Let mixture boil, then continue cooking for five minutes. Turn heat down to medium-low and whisk in basil sprig and half-and-half. Cook for eight minutes, discard basil sprig, and stir in Parmesan, chopped basil, pepper, and salt.
- Serve chicken with sauce.

Turkey Breast with Lean Bolognese Sauce

Nutritional Facts (Meat): Calories 226 Fat 10.0 g Protein 32.5 g Carbohydrates 0 g

Nutritional Facts (Sauce): Calories 100 Fat 2.0 g Protein 9.0 g Carbohydrates 7.0 g

Prep Time: 40 min **Cook time:** 55 min

Servings: 10 (Meat), 12 (Sauce)

Ingredients:

Meat:

- Olive oil (1 tablespoon)
- Poultry seasoning, dry (1/2 tablespoon)
- Turley breast, bone in, skin on, w/ ribs removed (4 pounds)
- Kosher salt (2 teaspoons)

Sauce:

- Tomatoes, crushed (28 ounces)
- Onion, large, chopped (1 piece)
- Mushrooms, chopped (8 ounces)
- Italian seasoning (1 tablespoon)
- Basil/parsley, chopped (1/2 cup)
- Olive oil, extra virgin (1 tablespoon)
- Garlic cloves, minced (4 pieces)
- Ground turkey, lean (1 pound)
- Salt (1/2 teaspoon)

Directions:

- Rub oil (1/2 tablespoon) an all sides of turkey breast. Sprinkle all over with pepper and salt, then coat the skin side with remaining oil (1/2 tablespoon).
- Preheat air fryer at 325 degrees Fahrenheit.
- Air-fry chicken for thirty minutes on each side.
- Stir onion into oil heated on medium in a skillet. Cook for five minutes, then stir in Italian seasoning and garlic. After one minute of stirring, add mushrooms, turkey, and salt; cook for ten minutes. Turn heat up to medium-high before stirring in tomatoes; cook for five minutes. Finish by stirring in parsley.
- Serve and enjoy.

Accessory #2 - Instant Meat And Food Thermometer

Fast, Accurate and Easy to use, this versatile meat thermometer enables you to prepare perfect meals without slicing your food. Simply insert the long temperature probe into your food / liquid and get perfectly cooked food every single time

For more information about this accessory go to:

www.MillenniumPublishingLimited.com > Barbara Trisler > Air Fryer Accessories

Chicken Chimichangas

Nutritional Facts: Calories 270 Fat 14.0 g Protein 16.0 g Carbohydrates 19.0 g

Prep Time: 28 min *Cook time:* 7 min

Servings: 8

Ingredients:

- Tortillas, flour, 6-inch (8 pieces)
- Dei rotisserie chicken, shredded (2 cups)
- Green chiles, chopped (4 ½ ounces)
- Water (3 tablespoons)
- Butter, melted (2 tablespoons)
- Vegetable oil (2 teaspoons)
- Seasoning mix, chicken taco (1 packet)
- Refried beans (3/4 cup)
- Cheddar cheese, shredded (1 cup)

Directions:

- Preheat air fryer at 375 degrees Fahrenheit.
- Heat oil in a skillet on medium. Stir in chicken, water, and taco seasoning mix. Cook for four to five minutes.
- Mix together chiles and beans. Spread 3 tablespoons of this mixture in center of each tortilla, then top with chicken (1/4 cup) and cheese (2 tablespoons). Fold sides of each tortilla to enclose filling.
- Brush melted butter on surface of each tortilla before placing in air fryer basket. Cook for four minutes on one side, and three minutes on the other.

The Healthier Chicken Nuggets

Nutritional Facts: Calories 188 Fat 4.5 g Protein 25.0 g Carbohydrates 8.0 g

Prep Time: 12 min *Cook time:* 8 min

Servings: 4

Ingredients:

- Breadcrumbs, Italian seasoned, whole wheat (6 tablespoons)
- Black pepper (1/2 teaspoon)
- Kosher salt (1/2 teaspoon)
- Parmesan cheese grated (2 tablespoons)
- Chicken breasts, boneless, skinless, sliced into one-inch chunks (16 ounces)
- Olive oil (2 teaspoons)
- Panko (2 tablespoons)
- Cooking spray, olive oil

Directions:

- Preheat air fryer at 375 degrees Fahrenheit.
- Fill a bowl with olive oil, and another with panko, breadcrumbs, and Parmesan.
- Sprinkle pepper and salt all over chicken. Dip in olive oil before coating with breadcrumb mixture. Mist all over with cooking spray.
- Air-fry for four minutes on each side.

Delicious Chicken Parmesan

Nutritional Facts: Calories 251 Fat 9.5 g Protein 31.5 g Carbohydrates 14.0 g

Prep Time: 21 min **Cook time:** 9 min

Servings: 4

Ingredients:

- Butter, melted (1 tablespoon) OR olive oil (1 tablespoon)
- Breadcrumbs, seasoned, whole wheat (6 tablespoons)
- Marinara (1/2 cup)
- Chicken breast, halved, 8-ounce (2 pieces)
- Parmesan cheese, grated (2 tablespoons)
- Mozzarella cheese, reduced fat (6 tablespoons)
- Cooking spray

Directions:

- Preheat air fryer at 360 degrees Fahrenheit. Mist cooking spray onto air fryer basket.
- Mix together parmesan cheese and breadcrumbs in a small bowl.
- Fill another bowl with melted butter. Brush butter on chicken before dipping in breadcrumb mixture.
- Mist cooking spray onto chicken before placing in air fryer. Cook for six minutes. Top each piece with sauce (1 tablespoon) and shredded mozzarella (1 ½ tablespoons), and air-fry for another three minutes.

Blue Cheese and Chicken Rolls

Nutritional Facts: Calories 231.5 Fat 6.0 g Protein 20.0 g Carbohydrates 24.5 g

Prep Time: 15 min **Cook time:** 30 min

Servings: 8

Ingredients:

- Carrots, shredded, chopped (1/3 cup)
- Cream cheese, reduced fat, softened (2 ounces)
- Egg roll wrappers (16 pieces)
- Blue cheese, crumbled (1/2 cup)
- Chicken breasts, skinless, boneless, 8-ounce (2 pieces)
- Hot sauce (1/2 cup)
- Scallions, chopped (1/3 cup)
- Blue cheese dressing
- Cooking spray, olive oil

Directions:

- Fill slow cooker pot with chicken and cover with water/chicken broth. Cover and cook on high for four hours. Transfer onto a plate, without the liquid, and shred with a fork.

- Mix together hot sauce and cream cheese. Stir in shredded chicken, carrots, scallions, and blue cheese.
- Preheat air fryer to 370 degrees Fahrenheit.
- Lay out egg roll wrappers and mold into diamond shapes. Fill each with buffalo dip mixture (3 tablespoons) and roll tightly to form a cylinder.
- Coat all rolls with cooking spray and air-fry for eight to nine minutes.

Pork Recipes

Red Beans, Rice and Cajun Pork Chop Packets

Nutritional Facts: Calories 260 Fat 8.5 g Protein 21.0 g Carbohydrates 24.5 g

Prep Time: 25 min **Cook time:** 20 min

Servings: 8

Ingredients:

- Pork chops, boneless, 5-ounce (4 pieces)
- Chicken broth, reduced sodium (3/4 cup)
- Kidney beans, red, drained, rinsed (19 ounces)
- Hot sauce (1 teaspoon)
- Green onions, w/ greens & whites separated, sliced thinly (6 pieces)
- Tomatoes, fire roasted, diced, undrained (14 ½ ounces)
- Cajun seasoning (2 teaspoons)
- Instant white rice, uncooked (1 cup)
- Green bell pepper, medium, diced (1 piece)
- Butter, melted (2 tablespoons)

Directions:

- Preheat air fryer to 350 degrees Fahrenheit.
- Combine tomatoes with Cajun seasoning (1/2 teaspoon), hot sauce, and chicken broth. Stir in instant rice and let sit for eight minutes. Stir in green onion whites, beans, and bell pepper.
- Brush melted butter all over pork chops. Rub with Cajun seasoning (1 ½ teaspoons) before placing each piece in a sheet of foil. Surround with rice-veggie mixture and sprinkle with remaining liquid.
- Seal all foil packets and add to the air fryer. Cook for thirty to thirty-five minutes.

Asian Pork and Edamame Dinner

Nutritional Facts: Calories 380 Fat 18.0 g Protein 34.0 g Carbohydrates 21.0 g

Prep Time: 20 min **Cook time:** 35 min

Servings: 4

Ingredients:

- Green onions, sliced thinly on the diagonal (2 pieces)
- Soy sauce (2 tablespoons)
- Lime juice, fresh (2 tablespoons)
- Butter, melted (3 tablespoons)
- Carrots, medium, peeled, sliced into ¾-inch chunks (4 pieces)
- Brown sugar, packed (2 tablespoons)
- Chili garlic sauce (1 tablespoon)
- Cilantro leaves, fresh, chopped (1/4 cup)
- Pork tenderloin, trimmed (1 pound)
- Shelled edamame, frozen, thawed (10 ounces)

Directions:

- Preheat air fryer to 375 degrees Fahrenheit.
- Mist cooking spray onto a rimmed sheet pan.
- Combine soy sauce and melted butter; toss with carrots. Place mixture on sheet pan and toss with pork. Spread into an even layer and top with remaining butter mixture.
- Air-fry for twenty-five minutes.
- Combine lime juice, chili garlic sauce, and brown sugar. Add edamame to pork and veggie mixture and drizzle with prepared sauce. Air-fry for eight minutes.

Prune Sauce Smothered Pork

Nutritional Facts: Calories 320 Fat 13.0 g Protein 27.0 g Carbohydrates 24.0 g

Prep Time: 30 min **Cook time:** 60 min

Servings: 12

Ingredients:

- Rice wine vinegar (1/4 cup)
- Kosher salt, coarse (1 teaspoon)
- Garlic clove, peeled (1 piece)
- Hot water (1 cup)
- Marjoram leaves, dried (1/2 teaspoon)
- Dinner roll, sourdough, 2-ounce, halved (1 piece)
- Guajillo chiles, dried, w/ seeds & stems removed (2 pieces)
- Plum tomatoes, halved (4 pieces)
- Tomato bouillon, w/ chicken flavor, granulated (1 teaspoon)
- Pork loin roast, rolled, boneless, 3-pound (1 piece)
- Olive oil (3 tablespoons)
- Onion, medium, chopped into 4 portions (1/2 piece)
- Chicken broth (2 ½ cups)
- Ancho chiles, dried, w/ seeds & stems removed (2 pieces)
- Plums, dried, pitted (2 cups)
- Thyme leaves, dried (1/2 teaspoon)
- Salt (1/2 teaspoon)

Directions:

- Preheat air fryer to 325 degrees Fahrenheit.
- Season pork roast with kosher salt (1 teaspoon).
- Heat oil (2 tablespoons) in roasting pan; add pork and cook for two minutes on each side. Transfer pork to plate and add oil (1 tablespoon) to same pan. Add onion, garlic, and dinner roll halves to cook for one minute. Transfer to a blender.
- Add pork back to pan and cover with broth (1/2 cup). Air-fry for ten minutes. Cover with foil and air-fry again for twenty-five minutes.

- Soak chiles for fifteen minutes in hot water. Drain and add to rolls mixture in blender. Add dried plums, thyme, salt (1/2 teaspoon), vinegar, tomatoes, marjoram, bouillon, and chicken broth (2 cups). Process until smooth, then pour into a saucepan and cook for ten minutes on medium heat.
- Smother pork with sauce mixture before air-frying for another twenty minutes. Serve with sauce.

Balsamic Blueberry Pork Delight

Nutritional Facts: Calories 267.3 Fat 6.1 g Protein 35.8 g Carbohydrates 14.4 g

Prep Time: 20 min *Cook time:* 40 min

Servings: 4

Ingredients:

- Black pepper (1 teaspoon)
- Garlic, minced (2 teaspoons)
- Garlic powder (2 teaspoons)
- Balsamic vinegar (1/2 cup)
- Pork tenderloin (1 ½ pounds)
- Salt (1 teaspoon)
- Blueberries, fresh/frozen (1/2 cup)
- Honey (1 tablespoon)

Directions:

- Preheat air fryer to 350 degrees Fahrenheit.
- Use aluminum foil to line baking sheet.
- Combine garlic powder, pepper, and salt. Rub all over pork. Place pork on sheet, mist all over with cooking spray, and air-fry for twenty to thirty minutes.
- Place blueberries in saucepan. Heat on medium and cook for two minutes. Stir in honey and garlic. Let mixture boil before stirring in balsamic vinegar. Let mixture boil again, then cook on simmer for twelve to fifteen minutes.
- Let pork sit on a plate for ten minutes. Slice into one-inch-medallions and cover with sauce.

Bacon Pork and Rainbow Veggies

Nutritional Facts: Calories 245 Fat 11.5 g Protein 20.5 g Carbohydrates 15.5 g

Prep Time: 10 min *Cook time:* 30 min

Servings: 12

Ingredients:

- Bacon, fatty (1 pound)
- Baby bella mushrooms, sliced in half (4 ounces)
- Red onions, large, chopped (2 pieces)
- Butternut squash, small, peeled, diced (1 piece)
- Cherry tomatoes (2 cups)
- Yellow bell peppers, large, sliced (2 pieces)
- Broccoli heads, chopped into florets (2 pieces)
- Olive oil (1/4 cup)

- Pork tenderloin (1 ½ pounds)
- Salt (1/4 teaspoon)
- Pepper (1/4 teaspoon)

Directions:

- Preheat air fryer to 425 degrees Fahrenheit.
- Place tomatoes, peppers, broccoli, mushrooms, red onions, and squash on sheet pan. After drizzling with olive oil, sprinkle with pepper and salt.
- Top bacon slices with pork. Sprinkle with pepper and salt before wrapping bacon around pork. Add on top of veggies and mist all over with cooking spray. Air-fry for twenty-five to thirty minutes.
- Let sit for five to ten minutes. Slice and serve along with veggies.

Tomato Pepper Pork Sandwiches

Nutritional Facts: Calories 430 Fat 17.0 g Protein 28.0 g Carbohydrates 42.0 g

Prep Time: 15 min **Cook time:** 45 min

Servings: 4

Ingredients:

Jam:

- Sugar (1/4 cup)
- Serrano pepper, seeded, diced (1 piece)
- Kosher salt (1/2 teaspoon)
- Grape tomatoes, quartered (1/2 pound)
- Red pepper, chopped (1/2 piece)
- Lemon juice (1 tablespoon)

Seasoning:

- Garlic powder (2 teaspoons)
- Kosher salt (1 teaspoon)
- Thyme, dried (1 teaspoon)
- Cayenne powder, dried (1/2 teaspoon)
- Paprika (1 tablespoon)
- Onion powder (2 teaspoons)
- Black pepper (1 teaspoon)
- Oregano, dried (1/2 teaspoon)

Sandwiches:

- Olive oil (2 tablespoons)
- Arugula (1 cup)
- Pork chops, medium, boneless (4 pieces)
- Sandwich buns (4 pieces)
- Red onions, sliced

Directions:

- Preheat air fryer to 325 degrees Fahrenheit.
- Heat tomato jam ingredients in a saucepan and let simmer for twenty minutes.
- Mix seasoning ingredients and rub all over pork chops. Mist all over with cooking spray. Air-fry for twenty minutes on each side. Let sit for five minutes, then slice into strips.

- Assemble sandwiches by topping buns' bottom halves with greens, onions, and pork chop strips. Serve garnished with tomato pepper jam.

Honeyed Ham Bake

Nutritional Facts: Calories 200 Fat 7.0 g Protein 26.0 g Carbohydrates 8.0 g

Prep Time: 10 min **Cook time:** 2 hrs 40 min

Servings: 12

Ingredients:

- Mustard, ground (1/2 teaspoon)
- Ham, bone in, smoked, fully cooked (6 pounds)
- Honey (1/4 cup)
- Cloves, ground (1/4 teaspoon)
- Cloves, whole

Directions:

- Preheat air fryer at 300 degrees Fahrenheit.
- Air-fry ham for twelve to sixteen minutes.
- Remove ham from air fryer and trim out uniform diamond shapes from its fat surface. Fill each diamond with a whole clove before brushing a mixture of ground cloves, honey, and mustard all over ham. Air-fry for twenty minutes.
- Tent with foil and let sit for ten minutes before serving.

Honey Barbecue Pork Packets

Nutritional Facts: Calories 470 Fat 12.0 g Protein 35.0 g Carbohydrates 57.0 g

Prep Time: 30 min **Cook time:** 30 min

Servings: 4

Ingredients:

- Honey (1/4 cup)
- Carrots, baby cut, ready to eat, sliced lengthwise in half (1 cup)
- Pork rib, boneless (4 pieces)
- Green onions, medium, sliced (2 pieces)
- Barbecue sauce (1/2 cup)
- Cumin, ground (2 teaspoons)
- Corn, large, each sliced into 6 portions (2 ears)
- New potato wedges, cooked, refrigerated (2 cups)

Directions:

- Preheat air fryer to 350 degrees Fahrenheit.

- Arrange 1 pork chop, ¼ cup carrots, ½ cup potato wedges, and 3 pieces corn in individual foil sheets.
- Combine barbecue sauce, cumin, and honey. Brush mixture all over contents in packets.
- Seal all foil packets and add to the air fryer. Cook for thirty to thirty-five minutes.

Easy Tonkatsu Pork

Nutritional Facts: Calories 305 Fat 18.5 g Protein 14.5 g Carbohydrates 19.5 g

Prep Time: 30 min **Cook time:** 30 min

Servings: 8

Ingredients:

Sauce:

- Dijon mustard (1 teaspoon)
- Brown sugar, packed (2 tablespoons)
- Ketchup (1/4 cup)
- Soy sauce (1 tablespoon)
- Worcestershire sauce (1 teaspoon)

Slaw:

- Green onions, sliced thinly on the diagonal (2 pieces)
- Coleslaw mix, tricolor (14 ounces)
- Sesame dressing (3/4 cup)

Pork:

- Breadcrumbs, panko, plain, crispy (3/4 cup)
- Egg (1 piece)
- Canola oil (1 ½ cups)
- Flour, all purpose (2 tablespoons)
- Soy sauce (1 tablespoon)
- Pork loin chops, boneless, thin, trimmed, ¼-pound (4 pieces)
- White rice, cooked

Directions:

- Preheat air fryer to 350 degrees Fahrenheit.
- Combine sauce ingredients.
- Combine slaw ingredients.
- Fill one bowl with flour, another bowl with beaten egg mixed with soy sauce (1 tablespoon), and a third bowl with breadcrumbs. Coat pork chops with flour before sipping in egg mixture and covering with breadcrumbs. Mist all over with cooking spray.
- Add chops to air fryer and cook for twenty-five to thirty minutes. Serve with sauce and slaw.

Chimichurri Pork

Nutritional Facts: Calories 265 Fat 15.5 g Protein 19.0 g Carbohydrates 13.0 g

Prep Time: 30 min **Cook time:** 30 min

Servings: 8

Ingredients:

- Olive oil (1 tablespoon)
- Salt (1 ¼ teaspoons)
- Butter (6 tablespoons)
- Queso fresco, crumbled (1/4 cup)
- Parsley leaves, fresh, chopped (1/2 cup)
- Red pepper flakes, crushed (1/2 teaspoon)
- Paprika, smoked (1 teaspoon)
- Lime wedges (4 pieces)
- Lime juice (1 tablespoon)
- Garlic cloves, chopped finely (2 pieces)
- Oregano leaves, fresh, chopped (1 teaspoon)
- Pork tenderloin, 1 ¼-pound (1 piece)
- Chili powder (1 teaspoon)
- Sweet corn, fresh, w/ husks removed (4 ears)
- Cilantro leaves, fresh, chopped (2 tablespoons)
- Cooking twine, 10-inch (4 pieces)

Directions:

- Preheat air fryer to 350 degrees Fahrenheit.
- Combine pepper, salt (1/4 teaspoon), parsley, olive oil, oregano, garlic, and lime juice.
- Pound pork until half-inch-thick. Cover with parsley mixture, then roll up lengthwise and secure with water-soaked kitchen twine.
- Brush melted butter (2 tablespoons) all over pork roll before rubbing with a mixture of smoked paprika, chili powder, and salt (1/2 teaspoon). Air-fry for twenty-five to thirty minutes.
- Tent with foil for five minutes, then discard twine and slice.
- Coat corn with melted butter (4 tablespoons) before sprinkling with salt (1/2 teaspoon). Air-fry for five to ten minutes and top with cilantro and queso fresco.
- Serve pork alongside corn and topped with lemon wedges.

Accessory #3 – Cooking Racks

Extra cooking racks increase the available cooking surface area of your air fryer, allowing you to cook two or more types of food at once. **Tambee** offers a number of cooking rack options, including 7 and 8 inch basic racks to fit air fryers of different sizes. Interestingly, they also offer an egg steaming rack that allows you to make up to seven hardboiled eggs in your air fryer.

For more information about this accessory go to:

www.MillenniumPublishingLimited.com > Barbara Trisler > Air Fryer Accessories

Beef Recipes

Easy Beef Bourguignon Kabobs

Nutritional Facts: Calories 310 Fat 13.0 g Protein 40.0 g Carbohydrates 7.0 g

Prep Time: 45 min *Cook time:* 10 min

Servings: 4

Ingredients:

- Thyme leaves, fresh, chopped (1 teaspoon)
- Red wine vinegar (1 tablespoon)
- Butter, melted (2 tablespoons)
- Yellow onion, medium, sliced into wedged chunks (1 piece)
- Parsley leaves, fresh, chopped (1 tablespoon)
- Olive oil (2 tablespoons)
- Salt (1 ¼ teaspoons)
- Bacon slices, thick cut, 2-inch (12 pieces)
- Honey (1 tablespoon)
- Red wine, dry (1/2 cup)
- Garlic cloves, minced (2 pieces)
- Mushrooms, fresh, halved (1/2 pound)
- Beef steak, top sirloin, boneless, cubed (1 ½ pounds)
- Sage leaves, fresh, chopped (1 teaspoon)
- Skewers, bamboo, 10-inch (8 pieces)

Directions:

- Preheat air fryer at 390 degrees Fahrenheit.
- Combine olive oil with honey and vinegar.
- Toss onion wedges and mushrooms with a mixture of melted butter, salt, wine, and garlic. Alternately thread onion and mushrooms onto 4 skewers.
- Coat beef with remaining wine mixture, then alternately thread with bacon on other 4 skewers.
- Air-fry for ten to twelve minutes. Serve sprinkled with sage, thyme, and parsley.

Double Decker Tacos

Nutritional Facts: Calories 290 Fat 10.0 g Protein 19.0 g Carbohydrates 30.0 g

Prep Time: 15 min *Cook time:* 5 min

Servings: 6

Ingredients:

- Chicken/beef (2 cups)
- Taco shells, hard (6 pieces)
- Tortillas, soft (6 pieces)
- Refried beans, heated (1 can)
- Toppings: salsa, sour cream, diced avocado, cheese, etc.

Directions:

- Preheat air fryer to 325 degrees Fahrenheit.

- Spread the top of each tortilla with refried beans (2 tablespoons) and then wrap around a taco shell.
- Mist cooking spray onto filled taco shells and tortillas. Air-fry for five minutes, turning halfway.
- Serve and enjoy.

Tasty Taco Cupcakes

Nutritional Facts: Calories 270 Fat 9.0 g Protein 12.0 g Carbohydrates 35.0 g

Prep Time: 10 min *Cook time:* 20 min

Servings: 18

Ingredients:

- Wonton wrappers (36 pieces)
- Taco seasoning mix (1 ounce)
- Tortilla chips (36 pieces)
- Ground beef (1 pound)
- Water (2/3 cup)
- Refried beans (16 ounces)
- Cheddar cheese, shredded (2 cups)
- Toppings: cilantro, sour cream, onion, diced tomatoes

Directions:

- Preheat air fryer to 350 degrees Fahrenheit. Mist cooking spray onto 18 muffin cups.
- Cook beef in skillet until browned; drain fat before adding water and taco seasoning mix. Let simmer for four to five minutes.
- Fill each muffin cup with a wonton wrapper. Fill each wrapper with refried beans (1 tablespoon), then top with crushed tortilla chip (1 piece), taco meat (1 tablespoon), and shredded cheese (1 tablespoon).
- Air-fry for fifteen to eighteen minutes. Serve topped with desired toppings.

Mouthwatering Lasagna Cupcakes

Nutritional Facts: Calories 254.9 Fat 13.2 g Protein 16.0 g Carbohydrates 17.4 g

Prep Time: 15 min *Cook time:* 20 min

Servings: 12

Ingredients:

- Ricotta cheese (3/4 cup)
- Parmesan cheese, grated (1 ¾ cups)
- Pasta sauce, Muir Glen (1 cup)
- Ground beef (1/3 pound)
- Wonton wrappers (24 pieces)
- Mozzarella cheese, shredded (1 ¾ cups)
- Basil
- Salt
- Pepper

Directions:

- Preheat air fryer to 350 degrees Fahrenheit. Mist cooking spray onto a muffin tin.
- Cook beef in skillet until browned, then sprinkle with pepper and salt before draining.
- Cut 2 ¼-inch-wide circles out of wonton wrappers.
- Set aside ¾ cup each of mozzarella cheese and parmesan cheese.
- Press a wonton wrapper into each muffin cup. Top each with layered parmesan, ricotta, and mozzarella cheeses, then with meat mixed with pasta sauce. Finish each by topping with reserved parmesan cheese and mozzarella cheese.
- Air-fry for eighteen to twenty minutes. Let cool before serving garnished with basil.

Cheeseburger Minis

Nutritional Facts: Calories 280 Fat 14.0 g Protein 15.0 g Carbohydrates 23.0 g

Prep Time: 20 min *Cook time:* 25 min

Servings: 9

Ingredients:

- Dill pickle, diced (1 piece)
- White onion, diced (1/2 piece)
- Salt (1/4 teaspoon)
- Pepper (1/4 teaspoon)
- Roma tomatoes, diced (2 pieces)
- Ground beef, lean (1 pound)
- Pizza crust, classic, refrigerated (1 container)
- Cheddar cheese, grated (4 ounces)
- Butter
- Mustard
- Ketchup

Directions:

- Preheat air fryer to 350 degrees Fahrenheit.
- Cook onions in oil until softened. Stir in ground beef and cook until browned and broken up. Season with pepper and salt. Set aside.
- Grease a muffin tin with cooking spray before filling with 9 dough sheets (cut out from lightly rolled out pizza crust), pressing down to create crusts.
- Fill each crust with beef mixture, then air-fry for sixteen to eighteen minutes. Sprinkle with cheese and air-fry for another two to three minutes.
- Serve garnished with desired toppings.

Frisée Salami Salad

Nutritional Facts: Calories 120 Fat 9.0 g Protein 4.0 g Carbohydrates 8.0 g

Prep Time: 10 min *Cook time:* 30 min

Servings: 8

Ingredients:

- Frisée, torn (4 bunches)
- Beef salami slices, kosher, sliced into quarter-inch strips (6 ounces)
- Mustard, coarse grained (2 teaspoons)
- Garlic clove, minced (1 piece)
- Black pepper, coarsely ground (1/4 teaspoon)
- Olive oil, extra virgin (1/4 cup)
- Red onion, medium, sliced (1/2 piece)
- Sherry vinegar (1 tablespoon + 1/3 cup)
- Kosher salt (1/2 teaspoon)
- Grape tomatoes, halved (1 pint)

Directions:

- Preheat air fryer at 350 degrees Fahrenheit.
- Brush salami strips with oil. Place in baking pan and air-fry for fifteen minutes.
- Stir garlic and onion in same pan and air-fry for ten minutes. Stir in salt, mustard, pepper, and vinegar, and air-fry for five minutes.
- Toss tomatoes and frisée with vinegar mixture, then sprinkle on top with salami strips.
- Serve and enjoy.

Easy Tortilla Casserole

Nutritional Facts: Calories 265 Fat 12.5 g Protein 14.5 g Carbohydrates 24.0 g

Prep Time: 25 min **Cook time:** 40 min

Servings: 12

Ingredients:

- Onion, small, chopped (1 piece)
- Cheeseburger macaroni, prepared (1 package)
- Salsa, chunky, thick (1 cup)
- Cheddar cheese, shredded (1 ½ cups)
- Ground beef, lean (1 pound)
- Hot water (1 1/3 cups)
- Milk (1/2 cup)
- Flour tortillas, six-inch (6 pieces)

Directions:

- Preheat air fryer to 325 degrees Fahrenheit.
- Cook onion and beef in skillet heated on medium-high until browned. Stir in salsa, hot water, milk, sauce mix, and uncooked pasta. Let mixture boil, then simmer, covered, until pasta is tenderly cooked.
- Slice each tortilla in half.
- Cover bottom of a baking dish with beef mixture (2 cups), then top with 6 tortilla halves, cheese (3/4 cup), beef mixture (2 cups), and remaining tortilla halves, beef mixture, and finally cheese.
- Air-fry for thirty minutes.

Baked Salsa Beef

Nutritional Facts: Calories 212.5 Fat 11.5 g Protein 12.0 g Carbohydrates 15.5 g

Prep Time: 15 min *Cook time:* 25 min

Servings: 6

Ingredients:

- Salsa, chunky, thick (16 ounces)
- Milk (3/4 cup)
- Cheddar cheese, shredded (1 cup)
- Ground beef, lean (1 pound)
- Biscuit mix (2 cups)
- Green onion, medium, chopped (1 piece)

Directions:

- Preheat air fryer to 375 degrees Fahrenheit.
- Mist cooking spray onto a square pan.
- Cook beef until browned; drain before stirring in salsa, then spread in pan.
- Stir together biscuit mix, cheese, onion, and milk to form a soft dough. Drop 12 tablespoons of dough on top of beef mixture in pan.
- Air-fry for twenty-five minutes.

Steak and Philly Cheese Biscuit Bake

Nutritional Facts: Calories 255 Fat 14.0 g Protein 13.5 g Carbohydrates 17.5 g

Prep Time: 40 min *Cook time:* 40 min

Servings: 16

Ingredients:

- Green bell peppers, medium, sliced thinly into strips (2 pieces)
- Steak seasoning (1 tablespoon)
- Cheese blend, mozzarella & provolone, shredded (2 cups)
- Onions, sliced thinly (2 cups)
- Biscuits, refrigerated, flaky layers (16 1/3 ounces)
- Ground beef, lean (1 pound)
- Vegetable oil (1 tablespoon)
- Velveeta, original, cubed (8 ounces)
- Milk (1 cup)

Directions:

- Preheat air fryer to 325 degrees Fahrenheit.
- Mist cooking spray onto a baking dish.
- Cook beef mixed with steak seasoning until browned. Drain and set aside in a bowl.
- Wipe-clean skillet and fill with vegetable oil. Heat on medium-high, stir in bell peppers and onions. Cook until browned before adding to beef bowl.
- Melt together cubed cheese, milk, and shredded cheese (1 cup); stir until smooth.
- Separate and cut dough to form 6 portions out of each of 8 biscuits. Stir into melted cheese mixture. Add to beef mixture and mix well. Pour into baking dish and top with remaining shredded cheese (1 cup).
- Air-fry for thirty-two to thirty-six minutes.

Beefy Stroganoff Casserole

Nutritional Facts: Calories 360 Fat 20.0 g Protein 21.0 g Carbohydrates 24.0 g

Prep Time: 25 min **Cook time:** 45 min

Servings: 6

Ingredients:

- Nutmeg (1/2 teaspoon)
- Ground beef, lean (1 pound)
- Pepper (1/4 teaspoon)
- Garlic cloves, minced (2 pieces)
- Sour cream (8 ounces)
- Egg noodles, medium, uncooked (8 ounces)
- Mushrooms, whole, fresh, small, halved (12 ounces)
- Gravy mix, beef/pork (2 ounces)
- Water (2 1/ 2cups)
- Parsley, fresh, chopped (1/4 cup)

Directions:

- Preheat air fryer to 350 degrees Fahrenheit.
- Mist cooking spray onto a casserole.
- Follow package directions in cooking egg noodles. Drain and keep warm by covering.
- Cook beef, garlic, and mushrooms until browned and fully cooked. Drain and set aside. Add to same skillet water, pepper, and gravy mix. Stir and cook until bubbling and thickened. Turn off heat before stirring in nutmeg and sour cream.
- Toss cooked noodles with gravy and beef mixture; add to casserole. Cover and air-fry for thirty to forty minutes.
- Serve sprinkled with parsley.

Seafood Recipes

Herb-Lemon Salmon Packets

Nutritional Facts: Calories 270 Fat 19.0 g Protein 23.0 g Carbohydrates 0 g

Prep Time: 15 min **Cook time:** 15 min

Servings: 4

Ingredients:

- Dill weed, fresh, chopped (1 tablespoon)
- Black pepper, ground (1/4 teaspoon)
- Lemon slices, thin (4 pieces)
- Butter, melted (4 tablespoons)
- Salt (1/2 teaspoon)
- Salmon fillets, skinless, 4-ounce (4 pieces)

Directions:

- Preheat air fryer at 350 degrees Fahrenheit.
- Prepare 4 individual foil sheets. Mist with cooking spray.
- Combine melted butter with pepper, salt, and dill weed. Toss with salmon.
- Fill each foil sheet with one fillet and half a slice of lemon. Twist and seal before placing on cookie sheet.
- Air-fry for fifteen to twenty minutes.

Vegetables and Shrimp Packets

Nutritional Facts: Calories 140 Fat 2.0 g Protein 17.0 g Carbohydrates 13.0 g

Prep Time: 5 min *Cook time:* 25 min

Servings: 2

Ingredients:

- Vegetables, antioxidant blend, frozen (7 ounces)
- Seasoning, old bay (2 teaspoons)
- Shrimp, 15-count, cleaned, shell on (1/2 pound)
- Lemon, thinly sliced (1/2 piece)

Directions:

- Preheat air fryer at 350 degrees Fahrenheit.
- Toss all ingredients until well-mixed. Divide mixture among 2 foil sheets. Top each with lemon slices and cover with another foil.
- Twist and seal foil packs and add to a cookie sheet.
- Air-fry for fifteen to twenty minutes.

Garlic Butter Shrimp Packets

Nutritional Facts: Calories 340 Fat 19.0 g Protein 22.0 g Carbohydrates 20.0 g

Prep Time: 10 min *Cook time:* 20 min

Servings: 4

Ingredients:

- Olive oil (2 tablespoons)
- Parsley, fresh, chopped (1 cup)
- Shrimp, peeled, deveined, uncooked (1 pound)
- Garlic cloves, grated (2 pieces)
- Polenta, 1-pound, refrigerated, sliced into half-inch portions (1 roll)
- Salt (1/4 teaspoon)
- Pepper (1/4 teaspoon)
- Butter, melted (4 tablespoons)
- Lemon juice (1 tablespoon)

For serving:

- Lemon wedges
- Parsley, fresh, chopped

Directions:

- Preheat air fryer at 350 degrees Fahrenheit.
- Prepare 4 individual sheets of foil. Pull up sides to form into packets. Mist with cooking spray.
- Fill each foil sheet with polenta slices, season with pepper and salt, and sprinkle with olive oil.
- Toss shrimp with garlic, melted butter, lemon juice, and parsley. Stir in pepper, red pepper flakes, and salt. Add shrimp mixture to foil sheets filled with polenta, including liquid.
- Twist and seal foil packs and arrange on cookie sheet. Air-fry for fifteen to twenty minutes.

Lime-Sake Edamame and Shrimp Packets

Nutritional Facts: Calories 280 Fat 8.0 g Protein 29.0 g Carbohydrates 21.0 g

Prep Time: 30 min **Cook time:** 20 min

Servings: 4

Ingredients:

- Cilantro, fresh, chopped (1/4 cup)
- Soy sauce (2 tablespoons)
- Shrimp, extra large, peeled, deveined, uncooked (1 pound)
- Sesame oil, toasted (1 tablespoon)
- Green onions, w/ greens & whites separated, sliced thinly (4 pieces)
- Sake (1/4 cup)
- Honey (2 tablespoons)
- Chili garlic sauce (1 tablespoon)
- Edamame, shelled, frozen (10 ounces)
- Lime wedges (8 pieces)

Directions:

- Preheat air fryer at 350 degrees Fahrenheit.
- Prepare 4 individual sheets of foil. Pull up sides to form into packets. Mist with cooking spray.
- Combine honey, chili garlic sauce, soy sauce, toasted sesame oil, and sake. Toss in shrimp, green onion whites, and frozen edamame.
- Fill each foil sheet with mixture, then drizzle with juice from squeezed lime. Seal foil packs and arrange on cookie sheet. Air-fry for fifteen to twenty minutes.
- Open foil packs and serve topped with green onion greens, cilantro, and lime wedges.

Spicy Lemon Mini Crab Cakes

Nutritional Facts: Calories 100 Fat 7.0 g Protein 4.0 g Carbohydrates 4.0 g

Prep Time: 40 min **Cook time:** 10 min

Servings: 24

Ingredients:

Crab cakes:

- Green onions, sliced thinly, w/ greens & whites separated (2 pieces)
- Eggs, beaten (2 pieces)
- Breadcrumbs, crispy, plain panko (1 cup)
- Lump crabmeat, pasteurized, refrigerated, cleaned (1 pound)
- Mayonnaise (1/4 cup)
- Chili garlic sauce (5 teaspoons)
- Olive oil (2 tablespoons)

Dressing:

- Lemon juice (1 tablespoon)
- Garlic, minced (1 piece)
- Mayonnaise (1/2 cup)
- Soy sauce (1 teaspoon)

Directions:

- Preheat air fryer to 390 degrees Fahrenheit.
- Mist cooking spray onto cookie sheet.
- Combine dressing ingredients, then cover and chill.
- Stir together crabmeat, mayonnaise (1/4 cup), chili garlic sauce, breadcrumbs, eggs, and green onion whites. Mold mixture into 24 patties. Cover and chill for ten minutes.
- Add patties to cookie sheet and brush all over with oil. Air-fry for ten to twelve minutes. Drain before serving topped with sauce and green onion greens.

Fontina Crab-Filled Mushrooms

Nutritional Facts: Calories 40 Fat 2.5 g Protein 2.0 g Carbohydrates 2.0 g

Prep Time: 30 min **Cook time:** 25 min

Servings: 24

Ingredients:

- Olive oil (1 tablespoon)
- Lump crabmeat, fresh (4 ounces)
- Lemon peel, grated (2 teaspoons)
- Butter, melted (1 tablespoon)
- Parmesan cheese, shredded (2 tablespoons)
- Salt (1/4 teaspoon)
- Baby bella mushrooms, washed, w/ stems removed (24 pieces)
- Breadcrumbs, crispy, plain panko (1/4 cup)
- Fontina cheese, shredded (3/4 cup)
- Green onions, chopped (2 tablespoons)
- Seafood seasoning mix (1 teaspoon)
- Dill weed, fresh, chopped (1 teaspoon)

Directions:

- Preheat air fryer at 375 degrees Fahrenheit. Mist cooking spray onto a pan.
- Toss mushrooms caps in olive oil before adding to pan. Air-fry for twelve minutes.
- Combine melted butter and breadcrumbs. Stir in fontina cheese, green onions, lemon peel, salt, Parmesan cheese, dill weed, seasoning, and crabmeat.

- Stuff mushroom caps with filling, then air-fry for another ten to twelve minutes.

Mediterranean Shrimp Skewers

Nutritional Facts: Calories 45 Fat 3.0 g Protein 3.0 g Carbohydrates 1.0 g

Prep Time: 45 min *Cook time:* 10 min

Servings: 24

Ingredients:

- Kalamata olives, pitted (24 pieces)
- Lemon juice (2 tablespoons)
- Olive oil (1 tablespoon)
- Feta cheese, cubed (8 ounces)
- Salt (1/2 teaspoon)
- Cherry tomatoes (24 pieces)
- Lemon peel, grated (1/2 teaspoon)
- Red pepper, crushed (1/2 teaspoon)
- Garlic cloves, minced (2 pieces)
- Shrimp, large, peeled, deveined, w/ tail shells removed, uncooked (24 pieces)
- Basil leaves, small (24 pieces)
- Cocktail skewers, 5-inch (24 pieces)

Directions:

- Preheat air fryer at 390 degrees Fahrenheit.
- Mist cooking spray onto a rimmed baking pan.
- Combine lemon juice, salt, oil, lemon peel, red pepper, and garlic. Toss in shrimp.
- Add shrimp mixture to pan and air-fry for ten to twelve minutes. Transfer to a bowl and chill for thirty minutes.
- Alternately thread cherry tomatoes, basil leaves (folded in half), shrimp head ends, olives, shrimp tail ends, and feta cheese cubes onto skewers.
- Serve and enjoy.

Sesame Shrimp Flatbread

Nutritional Facts: Calories 200 Fat 9.0 g Protein 11.0 g Carbohydrates 18.0 g

Prep Time: 15 min *Cook time:* 15 min

Servings: 10

Ingredients:

- Cilantro leaves, fresh, chopped (1/4 cup)
- Sesame oil, toasted (1 tablespoon)
- Carrots, shredded (1 cup)
- Soy sauce (1 tablespoon)
- Avocado, peeled, sliced thinly, sliced into thirds (1/2 piece)
- Pizza crust, thin, refrigerated (11 ounces)
- Shrimp, medium, peeled, deveined, w/ tail shells removed, uncooked (20 pieces)

- Mozzarella cheese, shredded (2 cups)
- Green onions, thinly sliced, w/ greens & whites separated (2 pieces)
- Sriracha sauce (1 tablespoon)

Directions:

- Preheat air fryer to 375 degrees Fahrenheit.
- Mist cooking spray onto cookie sheet. Press unrolled dough onto sheet and coat with sesame oil. Air-fry for eight to ten minutes.
- Toss shrimp with soy sauce.
- Spread on top of crust the following: cheese (1 cup), carrots, green onion whites, shrimp mixture, and cheese (1 cup).
- Air-fry for seven to eleven minutes. Serve topped with avocado, cilantro, and green onion greens, then drizzled with Sriracha.

Shrimp à la King

Nutritional Facts: Calories 290 Fat 7.0 g Protein 13.0 g Carbohydrates 45.0 g

Prep Time: 15 min **Cook time:** 10 min

Servings: 6

Ingredients:

- Skim milk (3/4 cup)
- Biscuit mix (2 ¼ cups + 1 tablespoon)
- Mixed vegetables, frozen (1 cup)
- Pepper (1/8 teaspoon)
- Clam chowder soup, prepared (18 ½ ounces)
- Salad shrimp, cooked, frozen, thawed, rinsed (5 ounces)
- Dill weed, dried (1 teaspoon)

Directions:

- Preheat air fryer at 425 degrees Fahrenheit.
- Combine milk and biscuit mix (2 ¼ cups) to form a soft dough. Drop 6 tablespoons, one tablespoon at a time, onto cookie sheet. Air-fry for ten minutes.
- Combine remaining ingredients in a saucepan and heat to boiling.
- Split each biscuit in half. Place each biscuit half on six individual plates, top with hot chowder mixture (1/4 cup), and cover with another biscuit half.
- Serve each filled biscuit topped with chowder mixture (1/4 cup).

Splendid Seafood Tartlets

Nutritional Facts: Calories 35 Fat 1.5 g Protein 2.0 g Carbohydrates 3.0 g

Prep Time: 10 min **Cook time:** 5 min

Servings: 30

Ingredients:

- Shrimp, tiny, rinsed, patted dry (30 pieces)
- Artichoke hearts, marinated, drained, chopped finely (6 ½ ounces)
- Seafood seasoning (1/2 teaspoon)
- Salad dressing/mayonnaise (2 tablespoons)
- Phyllo dough shells, mini, frozen (30 pieces)
- Lump crabmeat, drained (6 ½ ounces)
- Cream cheese spread, onion & chive (1/4 cup)
- Red onion, chopped (2 tablespoons)
- Parsley sprigs, fresh

Directions:

- Preheat air fryer at 375 degrees Fahrenheit.
- Arrange dough shells on cookie sheet. Mist all over with cooking spray. Air-fry for five minutes.
- Combine crabmeat, cream cheese spread onion, seafood seasoning, artichoke hearts, and mayonnaise.
- Fill each shell with crabmeat mixture (1 tablespoon). Serve tartlets garnished with parsley and thyme.

Accessory #4 – Parchment Liners

Some foods, especially those with a flour or breadcrumb coating, are known to stick to the bottom of the Air Fryer. Using this parchment liner will make the clean up so much easier!

For more information about this accessory go to:

www.MillenniumPublishingLimited.com > Barbara Trisler > Air Fryer Accessories

Vegetable Recipes

Cheesy Vegetable Fiesta Pie

Nutritional Facts: Calories 330 Fat 19.0 g Protein 16.0 g Carbohydrates 26.0 g

Prep Time: 15 min *Cook time:* 1 hr 20 min

Servings: 6

Ingredients:

- Eggs (2 pieces)
- Water, hot (4 cups)
- Jalapeno chiles, small, seeded, chopped finely (2 pieces)
- Salt (1/2 teaspoon)
- Egg, slightly beaten (1 piece)
- Flour, all purpose (2 tablespoons)
- Hash brown potatoes, prepared (1 box)
- Butter, melted (2 tablespoons)
- Cheese, Colby-Monterey Jack, shredded (2 cups)
- Red bell pepper, small, chopped finely (1 piece)
- Milk (2/3 cup)
- Sour cream
- Lettuce, shredded
- Chile peppers, sliced

Directions:

- Preheat air fryer at 350 degrees Fahrenheit.
- Soak potatoes in water and let stand for fifteen minutes. Drain and toss with egg and melted butter. Press mixture into a pie plate and air-fry for twenty minutes.
- Reduce air fryer temperature to 325 degrees Fahrenheit.
- Top potato crust with ½ of cheese, bell pepper, and chiles, then remaining ½ cheese, bell pepper, and chiles. Cover with beaten mixture of 2 eggs, flour, milk, and salt.
- Air-fry for thirty-five minutes. Slice and serve garnished with sour cream, chile peppers, and lettuce.

Sour Cream Squash Casserole

Nutritional Facts: Calories 253 Fat 18.0 g Protein 9.0 g Carbohydrates 16.0 g

Prep Time: 30 min *Cook time:* 50 min

Servings: 12

Ingredients:

- Buttery crackers, round, crushed (2 cups)
- Onion, large, chopped (1 piece)
- Soup mix, savory herb & garlic (1 teaspoon)
- Sour cream (8 ounces)
- Salt (1/2 teaspoon)
- Butter (6 tablespoons)
- Summer squash, yellow, sliced (4 pounds)
- Italian cheese blend, shredded (2 cups)
- Eggs (2 pieces)

Directions:

- Preheat air fryer at 325 degrees Fahrenheit.
- Mist cooking spray onto a baking dish.
- Cook onion in melted butter (2 tablespoons) for three minutes. Stir in squash and cook for ten minutes. Turn off heat before stirring in cheese, eggs, salt, soup mix, and sour cream.
- Melt butter (1/4 cup) and mix with crushed crackers. Sprinkle on dish and air-fry for forty minutes.

Heavenly Collard Bread

Nutritional Facts: Calories 300 Fat 15.0 g Protein 12.0 g Carbohydrates 29.0 g

Prep Time: 45 min ***Cook time:*** 40 min

Servings: 8

Ingredients:

Bread:

- Milk (1/2 cup)
- Red bell pepper, chopped (1/2 cup)
- Seasoned salt (1 teaspoon)
- Eggs (3 pieces)
- Red pepper flakes, crushed (1 teaspoon)
- Collard greens, chopped, frozen, thawed, drained (4 cups)
- Green onions, chopped (1/2 cup)
- Flour, all purpose (3 tablespoons)
- Cheddar cheese, shredded (1 cup)

Topping:

- Red bell pepper, chopped (1/2 cup)
- Butter, melted (2 tablespoons)
- Corn, whole kernel, drained (1/2 cup)
- Egg (1 piece)
- Muffin & cornbread mix (6 ½ ounces)
- Green onions, sliced (1/2 cup)
- Milk (1/3 cup)
- Red pepper flakes, crushed (1/2 teaspoon)

Directions:

- Preheat air fryer at 325 degrees Fahrenheit.
- Mist cooking spray onto a baking dish.
- Toss collard greens with green onions and bell pepper.
- Stir eggs and milk with seasoned salt and flour. Stir in collard mixture, cheese, and crushed red pepper (1 teaspoon). Spread into baking dish and air-fry for twenty-five minutes.
- Combine topping ingredients and spread over dish. Air-fry for thirty-five to forty minutes. Let cool before slicing into 8 portions.

Tasty Tomato Ziti Dish

Nutritional Facts: Calories 320 Fat 7.0 g Protein 19.0 g Carbohydrates 45.0 g

Prep Time: 30 min ***Cook time:*** 25 min

Servings: 6

Ingredients:

- Pepper (1/4 teaspoon)
- Burgers, soy protein, frozen, thawed, chopped finely (4 pieces)
- Tomato sauce, canned (15 ounces)
- Mozzarella cheese, shredded (3/4 cup)
- Garlic cloves, chopped finely (2 pieces)
- Oregano leaves, fresh, chopped (2 teaspoons)
- Ziti pasta, uncooked (2 ½ cups)
- Sweet onion, large, chopped (1 piece)
- Zucchini, medium, sliced lengthwise into ¼-inch-thick halves (1 piece)
- Tomatoes, fire roasted, diced, drained (14 ½ ounces)
- Salt, kosher/sea (1/4 teaspoon)

Directions:

- Preheat air fryer at 350 degrees Fahrenheit.
- Follow package directions in cooking and draining pasta.
- Mist cooking spray onto a baking dish.
- In skillet heated on medium, cook onion, garlic, and burgers until browned and cooked through. Stir in zucchini and cook for two minutes. Stir in tomatoes, salt, pepper, oregano, and tomato sauce. Let mixture boil, then toss in pasta. Pour into baking dish.
- Cover and air-fry for twenty minutes. Uncover and top with cheese. Air-fry for another five minutes.

Cheddar Cauliflower Pops

Nutritional Facts: Calories 120 Fat 9.0 g Protein 5.0 g Carbohydrates 6.0 g

Prep Time: 10 min **Cook time:** 25 min

Servings: 3

Ingredients:

- Olive oil (1 tablespoon)
- Black pepper (1/8 teaspoon)
- Cauliflower florets, small (3 cups)
- Salt (1/4 teaspoon)
- Cheddar cheese, sharp, shredded finely (1/3 cup)

Directions:

- Preheat air fryer at 425 degrees Fahrenheit.
- Toss cauliflower with oil, pepper, and salt. Add to a baking pan and air-fry for eighteen to twenty-two minutes, tossing halfway.
- Top with cheese and serve right away.

Chili Pepper Casserole

Nutritional Facts: Calories 170 Fat 4.5 g Protein 9.0 g Carbohydrates 23.0 g

Prep Time: 20 min **Cook time:** 30 min

Servings: 2

Ingredients:

- Salsa, reduced sodium (1/4 cup)
- Bulgur, uncooked (2 tablespoons)
- Marjoram leaves, dried (1/4 teaspoon) OR marjoram, fresh, chopped (1 teaspoon)
- Mozzarella cheese, reduced fat, shredded (1/3 cup)
- Chile pepper, whole, roasted (8 ounces)
- Boiling water (1/3 cup)
- Corn, whole kernel, frozen, thawed (1/3 cup)
- Jalapeno pepper, fresh, chopped (1/2 teaspoon)
- Garlic powder (1/4 teaspoon)
- Yogurt, fat free, plain (1/4 cup)

Directions:

- Preheat air fryer at 325 degrees Fahrenheit. Mist cooking spray onto a baking dish.
- Soak bulgur in water for ten minutes. Stir in cheese (1/4 cup), corn, garlic powder, jalapeno, and marjoram.
- Slice chiles and remove seeds and ribs. Drain and stuff each with filling (1/4 cup).
- Arrange stuffed chiles in baking dish and top with remaining cheese and salsa. Air-fry for twenty-five to thirty minutes. Serve each topped with a dollop of yogurt.

Sweet Pepper Poppers

Nutritional Facts: Calories 110 Fat 7.0 g Protein 5.0 g Carbohydrates 7.0 g

Prep Time: 30 min **Cook time:** 35 min

Servings: 16

Ingredients:

- Sweet peppers, mini, red/orange/yellow, sliced lengthwise in two, seeded (16 pieces)
- Heavy whipping cream (2 tablespoons)
- Salt (1/4 teaspoon)
- Butter, melted (2 tablespoons)
- Garlic clove, chopped finely (1 piece)
- Parmesan cheese, shredded (1/4 cup)
- Chevre cheese (8 ounces)
- Green onions, sliced thinly (1/4 cup)
- Red pepper flakes, crushed (1/2 teaspoon)
- Breadcrumbs, panko, plain, crispy (1/2 cup)
- Thyme leaves, fresh, chopped (1 teaspoon)

Directions:

- Preheat air fryer at 325 degrees Fahrenheit.

- Mist cooking spray onto a cookie sheet.
- Heat whipped cream and goat cheese in microwave to soften, then stir together with salt, garlic, green onions, and pepper flakes.
- Combine breadcrumbs, melted butter, and parmesan cheese.
- Fill pepper halves with goat cheese mixture. Sprinkle on top with breadcrumbs and arrange on cookie sheet. Air-fry for thirty to thirty-four minutes.
- Serve sprinkled with thyme.

Corn-Stuffed Jalapeno Poppers

Nutritional Facts: Calories 100 Fat 7.0 g Protein 2.0 g Carbohydrates 6.0 g

Prep Time: 25 min *Cook time:* 35 min

Servings: 16

Ingredients:

- Black beans, canned, drained, rinsed (1/2 cup)
- Butter, melted (2 tablespoons)
- Breadcrumbs, panko, crispy, plain (1/2 cup)
- Cilantro leaves, fresh, chopped (1 tablespoon)
- Cream cheese, softened (8 ounces)
- Sweet corn, whole kernel, frozen, thawed, drained (1/2 cup)
- 4-cheese blend, Mexican, shredded finely (1/4 cup)
- Jalapeno chiles, medium, halved lengthwise, seeded (8 pieces)

Directions:

- Preheat air fryer at 325 degrees Fahrenheit.
- Mist cooking spray onto a cookie sheet.
- Combine beans, corn, and cream cheese.
- Combine breadcrumbs, melted butter, and Mexican cheese blend.
- Fill jalapeno halves with cream cheese and arrange on cookie sheet. Top with breadcrumb mixture and air-fry for twenty-eight to thirty-two minutes.
- Serve sprinkled with cilantro.

Garlic Butter Potato Skins with Artichoke-Spinach Dip

Nutritional Facts: Calories 140 Fat 7.0 g Protein 5.0 g Carbohydrates 14.0 g

Prep Time: 40 min *Cook time:* 50 min

Servings: 20

Ingredients:

- Tomato, diced (1/2 cup)
- Cream cheese, softened (8 ounces)

- Baby spinach, chopped (1 cup)
- Red pepper flakes, crushed (1 teaspoon)
- Garlic cloves, peeled (3 pieces)
- Baby red potatoes (3 pounds)
- Parmesan cheese, shredded (5 ounces)
- Artichoke hearts, marinated, drained, chopped (6 ounces)
- Butter (2 tablespoons)
- Salt (1/4 teaspoon)

Directions:

- Preheat air fryer at 350 degrees Fahrenheit.
- Mist cooking spray onto a baking sheet. Fill with potatoes. Air-fry for forty-five minutes to one hour. Let cool before slicing into lengthwise halves. Scoop out flesh so you have 1/8-inch potato shells.
- Beat together cream cheese, pepper flakes, and parmesan cheese until well-mixed. Stir in spinach and artichoke hearts.
- In skillet heated on low, cook garlic cloves in melted butter for two to three minutes.
- Add potato skins to baking sheet and brush on top with garlic butter. Season with salt and air-fry for four to six minutes. Top with cream cheese mixture and air-fry for another one to two minutes.
- Serve topped with diced tomato.

Cheesy Basil Tomato Bruschetta

Nutritional Facts: Calories 80 Fat 6.4 g Protein 3.6 g Carbohydrates 2.0 g

Prep Time: 15 min **Cook time:** 40 min

Servings: 14

Ingredients:

- Parmesan cheese, shaved (1/2 cup)
- Olive oil (1/4 cup)
- Salt (1/2 teaspoon)
- Shallots, sliced into rings (2 pieces)
- Basil leaves, fresh, shredded (2 tablespoons)
- Baguette slices, half-inch-thick (14 pieces)
- Grape tomatoes (2 cups)
- Balsamic vinegar (1 tablespoon)
- Pepper (1/4 teaspoon)
- Basil leaves, fresh

Directions:

- Preheat air fryer at 400 degrees Fahrenheit.
- Arrange baguette slices on cookie sheet and brush with oil (2 tablespoons). Air-fry for six minutes.
- In a baking pan, toss shallots and tomatoes with a mixture of oil (2 tablespoons), pepper, salt, and vinegar. Air-fry for twenty-five minutes. Let cool.
- Combine shredded basil and tomato mixture, then spread over baguette slices. Serve topped with cheese and basil leaves.

Side Dishes

Easy Polenta Pie

Nutritional Facts: Calories 195 Fat 7.0 g Protein 10.0 g Carbohydrates 27.0 g

Prep Time: 10 min *Cook time:* 55 min

Servings: 6

Ingredients:

- Egg, slightly beaten (1 piece)
- Water (2 cups)
- Monterey Jack cheese, w/ jalapeno peppers, shredded (3/4 cup)
- Cornmeal (3/4 cup)
- Salt (1/4 teaspoon)
- Chili beans, drained (15 ounces)
- Tortilla chips/crushed corn (1/3 cup)

Directions:

- Preheat air fryer at 350 degrees Fahrenheit.
- Mist cooking spray onto a pie plate.
- In saucepan heated on medium-high, combine water, salt, and cornmeal. Let mixture boil, then cook on medium heat for six minutes. Stir in egg and let sit for five minutes.
- Pour cornmeal mixture into pie plate and spread evenly. Air-fry for fifteen minutes and top with beans, corn chips, and cheese. Air-fry for another twenty minutes.

Bean and Rice Dish

Nutritional Facts: Calories 440 Fat 6.0 g Protein 20.0 g Carbohydrates 77.0 g

Prep Time: 10 min *Cook time:* 1 hr 5 min

Servings: 4

Ingredients:

- Boiling water (1 ½ cups)
- Kidney beans, dark red, undrained (15 ounces)
- Marjoram leaves, dried (1/2 teaspoon)
- Cheddar cheese, shredded (1/2 cup)
- White rice, long grain, uncooked (1 cup)
- Bouillon, chicken/vegetable, granulated (1 tablespoon)
- Onion, medium, chopped (1 piece)
- Baby lima beans, frozen, thawed, drained (9 ounces)

Directions:

- Preheat air fryer at 325 degrees Fahrenheit.
- Combine all ingredients, save for cheese, in casserole.

- Cover and air-fry for one hour and fifteen minutes. Give dish a stir before topping with cheese.

Cheesy Potato Mash Casserole

Nutritional Facts: Calories 110 Fat 2.5 g Protein 4.0 g Carbohydrates 18.0 g

Prep Time: 25 min *Cook time:* 1 hr 10 min

Servings: 24

Ingredients:

- Chives, fresh, chopped (1 teaspoon)
- Cream cheese, reduced fat, softened (3 ounces)
- Yogurt, plain, fat free (1 cup)
- Cheddar cheese, reduced fat, shredded (1 cup)
- Paprika (1/4 teaspoon)
- White potatoes, peeled, cubed (5 pounds)
- Blue cheese, crumbled (1/4 cup)
- Parmesan cheese, shredded (1/4 cup)
- Garlic salt (1 teaspoon)

Directions:

- Place potatoes in saucepan filled with water. Heat to boiling, then cook on simmer for fifteen to eighteen minutes.
- Beat together parmesan cheese, cheddar cheese, cream cheese, and blue cheese until smooth. Beat in garlic salt and yogurt.
- Preheat air fryer t o 325 degrees Fahrenheit.
- Mash cooked potatoes until smooth. Stir in cheese mixture. Add to a baking dish and air-fry for thirty-five to forty minutes.

Simple Squash Casserole

Nutritional Facts: Calories 110 Fat 5.0 g Protein 4.0 g Carbohydrates 12.0 g

Prep Time: 20 min *Cook time:* 40 min

Servings: 6

Ingredients:

- Yellow summer squash, medium, sliced thinly (1 piece)
- Thyme leaves, fresh, chopped (1 tablespoon)
- Salt (1/2 teaspoon)
- Italian cheese blend, gluten free, shredded (1/2 cup)
- Olive oil, extra virgin (1 tablespoon)
- Zucchini, medium, sliced thinly (1 piece)
- Onion, diced (1/2 cup)
- Brown rice, cooked (1 cup)
- Plum tomato, diced (1 piece)
- Pepper (1/8 teaspoon)

Directions:

- Preheat air fryer to 375 degrees Fahrenheit.
- Mist cooking spray onto a gratin dish.
- Combine rice, onion, tomato, pepper, salt (1/4 teaspoon), oil, and ½ thyme leaves. Spread evenly into gratin dish and layer on top with squash and zucchini. Sprinkle with remaining salt (1/4 teaspoon) and thyme.
- Cover and air-fry for twenty minutes. Top with cheese and air-fry for another ten to twelve minutes.

Delicious Ginger Pork Lasagna

Nutritional Facts: Calories 480 Fat 24.0 g Protein 28.0 g Carbohydrates 37.0 g

Prep Time: 45 min **Cook time:** 45 min

Servings: 8

Ingredients:

- Thai basil leaves, fresh, sliced thinly (2 tablespoons)
- Butter (1 tablespoon)
- Garlic cloves, minced (2 pieces)
- Ricotta cheese, part skim (15 ounces)
- Wonton wrappers, square (48 pieces)
- Green onion greens & whites, separated, sliced thinly (4 pieces)
- Fish sauce (1 tablespoon)
- Parmesan cheese, shredded (1 tablespoon)
- Sesame oil, toasted (1 tablespoon)
- Ground pork (1 pound)
- Gingerroot, fresh, minced (1 tablespoon)
- Tomato sauce (15 ounces)
- Chili garlic sauce (1 tablespoon)
- Coconut milk (1/2 cup)

Directions:

- Preheat air fryer at 325 degrees Fahrenheit.
- Mist cooking spray onto a baking dish.
- In skillet heated on medium, cook pork in butter and sesame oil for eight to ten minutes. Stir in garlic, green onion whites, and gingerroot and cook for one to two minutes. Stir in fish sauce, chili garlic sauce, and tomato sauce. Cook on gentle simmer.
- Combine coconut milk, ricotta cheese, and parmesan cheese (1 cup).
- Arrange 8 overlapping wonton wrappers in baking dish to line bottom, then top with a second layer of eight wrappers. Spread on top 1/3 of cheese mixture, and layer with 1/3 of pork mixture. Repeat layering twice and finish by topping with parmesan cheese.
- Cover dish with foil and air-fry for thirty minutes. Remove foil and air-fry for another ten to fifteen minutes.
- Serve topped with basil and green onion greens.

Comforting Green Bean Casserole

Nutritional Facts: Calories 120 Fat 1.5 g Protein 7.0 g Carbohydrates 20.0 g

Prep Time: 30 min *Cook time:* 30 min

Servings: 8

Ingredients:

- Green beans, French cut, frozen, thawed, drained (16 ounces)
- Breadcrumbs, dry, plain (1/2 cup)
- Thyme, dried (1/2 teaspoon)
- Mushrooms, sliced (1/2 pound)
- Flour, all purpose (1/4 cup)
- Buttermilk (1/2 cup)
- Onion, cut into quarter-inch-thick rings (1 piece)
- Onion, small, chopped (1 piece)
- Salt (1/4 teaspoon)
- Milk, 1% (3 cups)

Directions:

- Preheat air fryer at 475 degrees Fahrenheit.
- Mist cooking spray into a baking dish and a baking sheet.
- Coat onion rings with buttermilk before covering with breadcrumbs and placing on baking sheet. Mist with cooking spray and air-fry for twenty minutes.
- Mist cooking spray onto a saucepan and heat on medium. Stir in chopped onion, salt, thyme, and mushrooms; mist with cooking spray and cook for four to five minutes. Stir in flour and cook for one minute. Stir in milk and cook for three to four minutes. Stir in green beans and remove from heat.
- Reduce air fryer temperature to 375 degrees Fahrenheit.
- Fill baking dish with bean mixture. Top with onion rings and air-fry for twenty-five to thirty minutes.

Fresh Veggie Tortellini

Nutritional Facts: Calories 180 Fat 9.0 g Protein 8.0 g Carbohydrates 20.0 g

Prep Time: 10 min *Cook time:* 15 min

Servings: 4

Ingredients:

- Plum tomatoes, chopped (2 cups)
- Olive oil (1 tablespoon)
- Italian seasoning (1/2 teaspoon)
- Tortellini, cheese filled, refrigerated (9 ounces)
- Bell pepper, medium, sliced into one-inch chunks (1 piece)
- Zucchini, medium, halved lengthwise, chopped into crosswise slices (1 piece)
- Garlic salt (1/2 teaspoon)

Directions:

- Follow package directions in cooking and draining tortellini. Set aside.

- In skillet heated on medium-high, stir bell pepper in olive oil and cook for two to three minutes. Stir in zucchini, tomatoes, garlic salt, and Italian seasoning; cook, covered, for three to five minutes. Toss in tortellini and cook for two to three minutes.
- Serve immediately.

Scrambled Basil and Potato

Nutritional Facts: Calories 120 Fat 0 g Protein 14.0 g Carbohydrates 18.0 g

Prep Time: 10 min *Cook time:* 20 min

Servings: 4

Ingredients:

- Eggs, large, beaten (8 pieces)
- Onion, minced (1/2 cup)
- Salt (1/2 teaspoon)
- White potatoes, medium, peeled, cubed (2 pieces)
- Red bell pepper, small, chopped (1 piece)
- Basil leaves, fresh, chopped (2 tablespoons)
- Red pepper, ground (1/8 teaspoon)

Directions:

- Preheat air fryer at 350 degrees Fahrenheit.
- In saucepan, cover potatoes with water and heat to boiling. Continue cooking, covered, on simmer for ten to fifteen minutes. Drain and toss with bell pepper and onion in a baking dish. Coat with cooking spray and air-fry for five to ten minutes.
- Combine all other ingredients and add to pan. Air-fry for three to five minutes.
- Serve right away.

Scrumptious Sweet Pea Wontons

Nutritional Facts: Calories 120 Fat 2.5 g Protein 3.0 g Carbohydrates 20.0 g

Prep Time: 20 min *Cook time:* 25 min

Servings: 40

Ingredients:

- Mint, fresh (2 tablespoons)
- Cream cheese, soft (8 ounces)
- Sweet peas (10 ounces)
- Eggs (2 pieces) mixed with water (2 tablespoons) to make egg wash
- Kosher salt (1/2 teaspoon)
- Wonton wrappers, square (40 pieces)

Directions:

- Preheat air fryer at 350 degrees Fahrenheit.
- Use parchment to line a baking sheet.
- Mash sweet peas together with salt and mint.
- Make egg wash by whisking eggs with water.
- Fill each wonton wrapper with cream cheese (1 teaspoon) and pea mixture (1 teaspoon), then fold up ends to form a triangle and seal by folding corners under.
- Brush egg wash on all filled wontons. Air-fry for fifteen to twenty minutes.

Onion Bread Pudding

Nutritional Facts: Calories 240 Fat 10.0 g Protein 14.0 g Carbohydrates 22.0 g

Prep Time: 35 min ***Cook time:*** 40 min

Servings: 12

Ingredients:

- Thyme leaves, dried (1 teaspoon)
- Sweet onions, large, diced (2 pieces)
- Eggs (4 pieces)
- Zucchini, shredded (3 cups)
- Salt (1 teaspoon)
- Olive oil (1 tablespoon)
- Rustic bread, whole grain, cubed (1 pound)
- Swiss cheese, shredded (2 cups)
- Milk (2 cups)
- Pepper (1/4 teaspoon)

Directions:

- Preheat air fryer at 325 degrees Fahrenheit.
- In skillet heated on medium-high, cook onions in oil for twenty to twenty-five minutes.
- Mist cooking spray into a baking dish. Fill with layered bread cubes (4 cups), zucchini (1 ½ cups), and cheese (3/4 cup); repeat layering once.
- Beat together all other ingredients and pour on top of bread mixture. Sprinkle with onions before covering with foil and air-frying for thirty to forty minutes. Top with cheese (1/2 cup) and air-fry for another two to three minutes.

Appetizers

Spanakopita Minis

Nutritional Facts: Calories 82 Fat 4.0 g Protein 4.0 g Carbohydrates 7.0 g

Prep Time: 25 min ***Cook time:*** 20 min

Servings: 8

Ingredients:

- Olive oil, extra virgin (1 tablespoon)
- Water (2 tablespoons)
- Egg white, large (1 piece)
- Salt, kosher (1/4 teaspoon)
- Feta cheese, crumbled (1 ounce)
- Oregano, dried (1 teaspoon)
- Phyllo dough, frozen, thawed (4 sheets)
- Baby spinach leaves (10 ounces)
- Cottage cheese, 1% low fat (1/4 cup)
- Parmesan cheese, grated finely (2 tablespoons)
- Lemon zest, freshly grated (1 teaspoon)
- Black pepper, freshly ground (1/4 teaspoon)
- Cayenne pepper (1/8 teaspoon)
- Cooking spray

Directions:

- Boil the spinach in a pot of water; once wilted, drain, cool, and pat-dry. Add to a bowl filled with egg white, feta cheese, cottage cheese, Parmesan cheese, black pepper, cayenne pepper, oregano, lemon zest, and salt; mix well.
- Brush the phyllo sheets with a little oil before stacking. Cut into 16 equal-sized strips. Add filling (1 tablespoon) onto one of each strip's end before folding the entire phyllo sheet into a triangular packet.
- Mist cooking spray onto the air fryer basket. Top with the packets, then mist again with cooking spray. Cook for twelve minutes at 375 degrees Fahrenheit.
- Serve right away.

Greek Feta Fries Overload

Nutritional Facts: Calories 383 Fat 16.0 g Protein 19.0 g Carbohydrates 42.0 g

Prep Time: 5 min **Cook time:** 40 min

Servings: 2

Ingredients:

- Potatoes, russet/Yukon gold, 7-ounce, scrubbed, dried (2 pieces)
- Salt, kosher (1/4 teaspoon)
- Black pepper, freshly ground (1/4 teaspoon)
- Plum tomatoes, seeded, diced (1/4 cup)
- Lemon zest, freshly grated (2 teaspoons)
- Onion powder (1/4 teaspoon)
- Chicken breast, rotisserie, skinless, shredded (2 ounces)
- Parsley, flat leaf, fresh, chopped (1/2 tablespoon)
- Oregano, fresh, chopped (1/2 tablespoon)
- Cooking spray
- Olive oil, extra virgin (1 tablespoon)
- Oregano, dried (1/2 teaspoon)
- Garlic powder (1/4 teaspoon)
- Paprika (1/4 teaspoon)
- Feta cheese, grated finely (2 ounces)
- Tzatziki, prepared (1/4 cup)
- Red onion, chopped (2 tablespoons)

Directions:

- Set the air fryer at 380 degrees Fahrenheit to preheat.
- Slice the potatoes into quarter-inch-thick fries. Add to a bowl filled with salt, pepper, onion powder, dried oregano, garlic powder, paprika, and zest, then toss until well-coated.

- Cook potato fries in the air fryer for fifteen minutes. Serve topped with feta cheese, shredded chicken, tzatziki, diced plum tomatoes, chopped red onion, and fresh herbs.

Sour Cream Mushrooms

Nutritional Facts: Calories 43 Fat 1.7 g Protein 2.4 g Carbohydrates 1.7 g

Prep Time: 30 min *Cook time:* 15 min

Servings: 24

Ingredients:

- Bell pepper, orange, diced (1/2 piece)
- Cheddar cheese, shredded (1 cup)
- Carrot, small, diced (1 piece)
- Cheddar cheese, shredded (1 ½ tablespoons)
- Mushrooms, w/ stems & caps diced (24 pieces)
- Onion, diced (1/2 piece)
- Bacon slices, diced (2 pieces)
- Sour cream (1/2 cup)

Directions:

- Sauté the onion, bacon, mushroom stems, carrot, and orange bell pepper. Once fully cooked, stir in sour cream and cheddar cheese (1 cup) and cook for two minutes.
- Set the air fryer at 350 degrees Fahrenheit to preheat.
- Fill mushroom caps with prepared stuffing before topping with remaining cheddar cheese.
- Cook in the air fryer for eight minutes or until cheese melts.

Tasty Zucchini Gratin

Nutritional Facts: Calories 82 Fat 5.2 g Protein 3.6 g Carbohydrates 6.1 g

Prep Time: 10 min *Cook time:* 15 min

Servings: 4

Ingredients:

- Parsley, fresh, chopped (1 tablespoon)
- Parmesan cheese, grated (4 tablespoons)
- Pepper, freshly cracked (1/4 teaspoon)
- Salt (1/4 teaspoon)
- Zucchini (2 pieces)
- Breadcrumbs (2 tablespoons)
- Vegetable oil (1 tablespoon)

Directions:

- Set the air fryer at 350 degrees Fahrenheit to preheat.
- Chop zucchini into 8 portions and add to the air fryer basket.
- Combine the breadcrumbs, black pepper, cheese, parsley, and oil. Add on top of the zucchini pieces.

- Cook for fifteen minutes.

Easiest Egg Rolls

Nutritional Facts: Calories 216 Fat 7.7 g Protein 10.6 g Carbohydrates 27.0 g

Prep Time: 30 min *Cook time:* 15 min

Servings: 16

Ingredients:

- Spinach, canned, drained (13 ½ ounces)
- Green onions, sliced (4 pieces)
- Salt (1 teaspoon)
- Cheddar cheese, sharp, shredded (1 cup)
- Cooking spray
- Egg roll, packaged (16 ounces)
- Corn, frozen, thawed (2 cups)
- Black beans, canned, drained, rinsed (15 ounces)
- Cheese, jalapeno Jack, shredded (1 ½ cups)
- Green chiles, canned, diced, drained (4 ounces)
- Cumin, ground (1 teaspoon)
- Chili powder (1 teaspoon)

Directions:

- Combine the filling ingredients: Cheddar cheese, jalapeno jack cheese, salt, chili powder, cumin, green onions, green chiles, spinach, and beans.
- Set the air fryer at 390 degrees Fahrenheit to preheat.
- Fill each egg roll wrapper with your filling. Fold, tuck, and mist with cooking spray.
- Add egg rolls to the air fryer and cook for eight minutes. Flip to cook for another four minutes.

Riced Cauliflower Balls

Nutritional Facts: Calories 257 Fat 11.5 g Protein 21.5 g Carbohydrates 15.6 g

Prep Time: 21 min *Cook time:* 9 min

Servings: 2

Ingredients:

- Cauliflower rice, frozen (2 ¼ cup)
- Egg, large, beaten (1 piece)

- Marinara, homemade (2 tablespoons)
- Cheese, parmesan/pecorino romano, grated (1 tablespoon)
- Chicken sausage, Italian, w/ casing removed (1 link)
- Salt, kosher (1/4 teaspoon)
- Cheese, mozzarella, part skim, shredded (1/2 cup)
- Breadcrumbs (1/4 cup)
- Cooking spray

Directions:

- Cook the sausage on medium-high until cooked through and broken up. Stir in the marinara, salt, and cauliflower and cook for another six minutes over medium heat. Turn off heat before stirring in the mozzarella.
- Spray the cooled cauliflower mixture with cooking spray before molding into 6 balls. Dip each ball in the beaten egg before coating with breadcrumbs. Load in the air fryer, coat with cooking spray, and cook for four to five minutes on each side at 400 degrees Fahrenheit.

All-Crisp Sweet Potato Skins

Nutritional Facts: Calories 150.5 Fat 6.0 g Protein 8.0 g Carbohydrates 25.0 g

Prep Time: 10 min **Cook time:** 50 min

Servings: 6

Ingredients:

- Scallions, sliced thinly (2 pieces)
- Cooking spray, olive oil
- Black beans, fat free, re-fried (1 cup)
- Salt, kosher (1/4 teaspoon)
- Cheese, cheddar, reduced fat, shredded (3/4 cup)
- Sweet potatoes, small (6 pieces)
- Taco seasoning (1/2 tablespoon)
- Black pepper, freshly ground (1/4 teaspoon)
- Salsa (3/4 cup)
- Cilantro, chopped (1 tablespoon)

Directions:

- Set the air fryer at 370 degrees Fahrenheit to preheat.
- Cover the sweet potatoes in parchment and cook in the air fryer for thirty minutes. Let cool.
- Mix together the taco seasoning and black beans.
- Halve the cooled sweet potatoes and remove most of the flesh. Spray the skins with cooking spray, sprinkle with pepper and salt, and air-fry for two to three minutes.
- Fill each skin with black beans, salsa (1 tablespoon), and cheese (1 tablespoon). Return to the air fryer and cook for two minutes.
- Serve topped with cilantro and scallions.

Korean-Style Chicken Wings

Nutritional Facts: Calories 451 Fat 19.0 g Protein 2.0 g Carbohydrates 44.0 g

Prep Time: 10 min *Cook time:* 30 min

Servings: 4

Ingredients:

- Cornstarch (3/4 cup)
- Onion powder (1 teaspoon)
- Chicken wings (2 pounds)
- Garlic powder (1 teaspoon)
- Salt (1/2 teaspoon)

Sauce:

- Soy sauce (1 tablespoon)
- Honey (3 tablespoons)
- Garlic, minced (1 teaspoon)
- Korean chili paste (2 tablespoons)
- Brown sugar (2 tablespoons)
- Salt (1/2 teaspoon)

Directions:

- Set the air fryer at 390 degrees F to preheat.
- Pat dry the chicken wings before seasoning with salt (1/2 teaspoon), garlic powder, and onion powder.
- Coat all seasoned chicken pieces with cornstarch and load in the air fryer. Cook for thirty minutes, turning halfway.
- Stir the sauce ingredients together and cook until boiling. Continue cooking on simmer for five minutes.
- Toss the wings with the sauce before serving.

Creamy Cauliflower Dip

Nutritional Facts: Calories 308 Fat 29.0 g Protein 7.0 g Carbohydrates 3.0 g

Prep Time: 10 min *Cook time:* 30 min

Servings: 10

Ingredients:

- Green onions, chopped (4 pieces)
- Olive oil, extra virgin (2 tablespoons)
- Worcestershire sauce (1 teaspoon)
- Mayonnaise (3/4 cup)
- Parmesan cheese, shredded (1 ½ cups)
- Cauliflower head (1 piece)
- Cream cheese, softened (8 ounces)
- Sour cream (1/2 cup)
- Garlic cloves (2 pieces)

Directions:

- Break the cauliflower into florets after washing and patting dry. Toss with olive oil until evenly coated.

- Place florets in the air fryer and cook for twenty minutes at 390 degrees Fahrenheit, turning halfway.
- Transfer the roasted florets into the blender and process with the sour cream, cream cheese, parmesan cheese (1 cup), mayonnaise, green onions, garlic, and Worcestershire sauce.
- Pour the blended cauliflower mixture into a bake dish (7x7-inch) and top with the remaining parmesan cheese. Cook in the air fryer for ten to fifteen minutes at 360 degrees Fahrenheit.

Chicken Bacon Bites

Nutritional Facts: Calories 339 Fat 16.0 g Protein 28.0 g Carbohydrates 18.0 g

Prep Time: 10 min *Cook time:* 13 min

Servings: 4

Ingredients:

- Bacon slices, cut into 1/3-portions (6 pieces)
- Chili powder (1/2 tablespoon)
- Chicken breast, sliced into one-inch chunks (1 pound)
- Brown sugar (1/3 cup)
- Cayenne pepper (1/8 teaspoon)

Directions:

- Stick a bacon piece onto a chicken piece, then roll to secure, finishing by piercing with a toothpick. Repeat with the remaining bacon and chicken pieces.
- Mix the brown sugar, cayenne pepper, and chili powder, then use to season the chicken bacon bites.
- Cook in the air fryer for fifteen minutes at 390 degrees F.

Snacks

Sweet Potato Bites

Nutritional Facts: Calories 78 Fat 0 g Protein 1.0 g Carbohydrates 19.0 g

Prep Time: 20 min *Cook time:* 60 min

Servings: 4

Ingredients:

- Potato starch (1 tablespoon)
- Salt, kosher, divided (1 ¼ teaspoons)
- Sweet potatoes, small, peeled (2 pieces)
- Ketchup, w/ no added salt (3/4 cup)
- Garlic powder (1/8 teaspoon)

- Cooking spray

Directions:

- Add sweet potatoes to a pot of boiling water. Cook for fifteen minutes, then let cool.
- After grating the sweet potatoes, combine with salt (1 teaspoon), garlic powder, and potato starch. Mold into one-inch cylinders.
- Apply cooking spray to the air fryer basket before filling with the sweet potato pieces. Cook for twelve to fourteen minutes at 400 degrees Fahrenheit.
- Sprinkle salt all over the sweet potato bites before serving.
- Enjoy right away with ketchup.

Chocolate-y! Churros

Nutritional Facts: Calories 173 Fat 11.0 g Protein 3.0 g Carbohydrates 12.0 g

Prep Time: 30 min **Cook time:** 55 min

Servings: 12

Ingredients:

- Sugar, granulated (1/3 cup)
- Salt, kosher (1/4 teaspoon)
- Baking chocolate, bittersweet, chopped finely (4 ounces)
- Butter, unsalted, divided (1/4 cup + 2 tablespoons)
- Vanilla kefir (2 tablespoons)
- Eggs, large (2 pieces)
- Water (1/2 cup)
- Flour, all purpose (1/2 cup)
- Cinnamon, ground (2 teaspoons)
- Heavy cream (3 tablespoons)

Directions:

- Combine the butter (1/4 cup) with salt and water. Let the mixture boil before stirring in the flour. Cook on a simmer until a smooth dough forms. Cook for another three minutes.
- Place cooked dough in a bowl. Give it a constant stir until a bit cool, then add one egg at a time as you keep stirring.
- Place the smooth batter in a piping bag and chill for half an hour.
- Pipe 3-inch-long churro-shaped pieces of the batter into the air fryer basket. Cook for ten minutes at 380 degrees Fahrenheit.
- Mix the cinnamon and sugar. Brush the remaining butter (2 tablespoons) all over the cooked churros before rolling in the cinnamon sugar.
- Melt the cream and chocolate in the microwave, then stir in the kefir.
- Serve churros drizzled with the chocolate sauce.

Nice 'n Crispy "Baked" Potatoes

Nutritional Facts: Calories 199 Fat 7.0 g Protein 7.0 g Carbohydrates 26.0 g

Prep Time: 10 min *Cook time:* 15 min

Servings: 2

Ingredients:

- Chives, fresh, chopped (1 ½ tablespoons)
- Olive oil, extra virgin (1 teaspoon)
- Sour cream, reduced fat (2 tablespoons)
- Baby potatoes, Yukon Gold (11 ounces)
- Bacon slices, center cut (2 pieces)
- Cheddar cheese reduced fat, shredded finely (1/2 ounce)
- Salt, kosher (1/8 teaspoon)

Directions:

- Preheat air fryer at 350 degrees Fahrenheit.
- Combine potatoes with oil until well-coated.
- Air-fry for twenty-five minutes. Place on platter and slightly crush to split.
- Cook bacon in skillet until crispy. Crumble and sprinkle over potatoes.
- Drizzle bacon drippings on top of potatoes before sprinkling with cheese, chives, sour cream, and salt.

Air-Fried Empanadas

Nutritional Facts: Calories 343 Fat 19.0 g Protein 17.0 g Carbohydrates 25.0 g

Prep Time: 30 min *Cook time:* 15 min

Servings: 2

Ingredients:

- Ground beef, 85% lean (3 ounces)
- Green olives, pitted, chopped (6 pieces)
- Tomatoes, chopped (1/2 cup)
- Cremini mushrooms, chopped finely (3 ounces)
- Cumin, ground (1/4 teaspoon)
- Egg, large, beaten lightly (1 piece)
- Olive oil, extra virgin (1 tablespoon)
- White onion, chopped finely (2 teaspoons)
- Garlic, chopped finely (2 teaspoons)
- Paprika (1/4 teaspoon)
- Cinnamon, ground (1/8 teaspoon)
- Gyoza wrappers, square (8 pieces)

Directions:

- Preheat air fryer at 400 degrees Fahrenheit.
- In skillet heated on medium-high, cook onion and beef in oil for three minutes. Stir in mushrooms and cook for six minutes. Stir in garlic, paprika, cinnamon, cumin, and olives. Cook for three minutes. Stir in tomatoes to cook for one minute. Place mixture in bowl and set aside.
- Fill each of 4 gyoza wrappers with filling (1 ½ tablespoons). Cover with egg-brushed edges of wrappers and pinch to seal.
- Air-fry for seven minutes.

Crunchy Calzones

Nutritional Facts: Calories 348 Fat 12.0 g Protein 21.0 g Carbohydrates 44.0 g

Prep Time: 15 min *Cook time:* 12 min

Servings: 2

Ingredients:

- Red onion, chopped finely (1/4 cup)
- Pizza dough, whole wheat, freshly prepared (6 ounces)
- Marinara sauce, reduced sodium (1/3 cup)
- Mozzarella cheese, part skim, pre-shredded (1 ½ ounces)
- Olive oil, extra virgin (1 teaspoon)
- Baby spinach leaves (3 ounces)
- Chicken breast, rotisserie, shredded (2 ounces)
- Cooking spray

Directions:

- Preheat air fryer at 325 degrees Fahrenheit.
- In skillet heated on medium-high, cook onion in oil for two minutes. Stir in spinach and cook until wilted. Turn off heat and stir in chicken and marinara sauce.
- Cut dough into 4 portions. Roll each piece into a six-inch round. Top each round with ¼ spinach mixture and ¼ cheese, then cover and seal with dough edges to form a half-moon.
- Mist cooking spray onto calzones before adding to air fryer. Cook for twelve minutes, turning halfway.

Butter-Lime Corn

Nutritional Facts: Calories 201 Fat 7.0 g Protein 6.0 g Carbohydrates 35.0 g

Prep Time: 10 min *Cook time:* 10 min

Servings: 4

Ingredients:

- Lime zest, freshly grated (1 teaspoon)
- Butter, unsalted (1 ½ tablespoons)
- Salt, kosher (1/2 teaspoon)
- Garlic, chopped (2 teaspoons)
- Cilantro, fresh, chopped (2 tablespoons)
- Corn, fresh, shucked (4 ears)
- Lime juice, freshly squeezed (1 tablespoon)
- Black pepper, freshly ground (1/2 teaspoon)
- Cooking spray

Directions:

- Preheat air fryer at 400 degrees Fahrenheit.

- Mist cooking spray onto corn before adding to air fryer basket. Cook for fourteen minutes, turning halfway.
- Combine melted butter, lime juice, garlic, and lime zest. Pour mixture on top of corn. Sprinkle with cilantro, salt, and pepper.
- Serve right away.

Crisp 'n Tender Sweet Potato Fries

Nutritional Facts: Calories 104 Fat 3.0 g Protein 1.0 g Carbohydrates 17.0 g

Prep Time: 10 min **Cook time:** 50 min

Servings: 4

Ingredients:

- Thyme, fresh, chopped (1 teaspoon)
- Garlic powder (1/4 teaspoon)
- Olive oil, extra virgin (1 tablespoon)
- Sweet potatoes, peeled, sliced into quarter-inch sticks (2 pieces)
- Sea salt, fine (1/4 teaspoon)
- Cooking spray

Directions:

- Toss sweet potato with mixture of salt, garlic powder, thyme, and olive oil.
- Preheat air fryer at 400 degrees Fahrenheit.
- Coat sweet potato with cooking spray. Air-fry for seven minutes on each side.

Buffalo Cauli Nuggets

Nutritional Facts: Calories 125 Fat 4.0 g Protein 5.0 g Carbohydrates 17.0 g

Prep Time: 10 min **Cook time:** 40 min

Servings: 4

Ingredients:

- Hot sauce (2 tablespoons)
- Sour cream, reduced fat (1/4 cup)
- Vinegar, red wine (1 teaspoon)
- Breadcrumbs, panko (3/4 cup)
- Blue cheese, crumbled (1 tablespoon)
- Black pepper, freshly ground (1/4 teaspoon)
- Ketchup, w/ no added salt (3 tablespoons)
- Egg white, large (1 piece)
- Cauliflower head, trimmed, sliced into one-inch florets (4 cups)
- Garlic clove, small, grated (1 piece)
- Cooking spray

Directions:

- Preheat air fryer at 320 degrees Fahrenheit.
- Whisk egg white with hot sauce and ketchup. Toss with cauliflower florets. Cover with panko, then coat with cooking spray.
- Air-fry for twenty minutes.
- Mix together blue cheese, pepper, garlic, vinegar, and sour cream.
- Serve buffalo cauli nuggets along with your blue cheese sauce.

Cheesy Vegan Chili Fries

Nutritional Facts: Calories 468 Fat 15.6 g Protein 18.9 g Carbohydrates 66.4 g

Prep Time: 30 min *Cook time:* 30 min

Servings: 4

Ingredients:

- Russet potatoes (25 ounces)
- Vegan chili
- Vegetable broth, hot (1/2 cup)
- Celery, diced (1/4 cup)
- Onion, diced (1/4 cup)
- Tomatoes, Mexican style, w/ green chiles, diced (10 ounces)
- Kidney beans, drained (1/3 cup)
- Chili powder, New Mexico (1 teaspoon)
- Salt, smoked (1/2 teaspoon)
- Pinto beans, drained (1/3 cup)
- Cumin, ground (1/2 teaspoon)
- Olive oil, extra virgin (1 tablespoon + 2 tablespoons)
- Vegetable protein, texturized (1/4 cup)
- Carrot, diced (1/4 cup)
- Garlic clove, minced (1 piece)
- Black beans, drained (1/3 cup)
- White beans, drained (1/3 cup)
- Blackstrap molasses (1/2 tablespoon)
- Oregano, Mexican, dried (1 teaspoon)
- Paprika, smoked (1/2 teaspoon)
- Black pepper, ground (1/2 teaspoon)
- Salt (1/4 teaspoon)
- Black pepper, freshly ground (1/4 teaspoon)

Cheese sauce:

- Soy milk, unsweetened (1/4 cup)
- Vegan cheese, cheddar-flavored, shredded (1/2 cup)
- Vegan butter (1 teaspoon)

Toppings:

- Jalapeno pepper, chopped into rings (1 piece)
- Red onion, minced (1/4 cup)
- Cilantro, minced (3 tablespoons)

Directions:

- Slice washed, unpeeled potatoes into shoestring pieces. Rinse under cool running water, then soak for thirty minutes in one inch of cold water.
- Soak texturized vegetable protein in hot vegetable broth.
- In a pot heated on medium, cook onion, celery, and carrot in olive oil (2 tablespoons). Stir in garlic, broth, and texturized vegetable protein, as well as drained beans, tomatoes, chili powder, cumin, smoked salt, pepper, oregano, paprika, and molasses. Simmer for fifteen minutes.
- Preheat air fryer at 320 degrees Fahrenheit.
- Drain and pat-dry potatoes and toss with olive oil (1 tablespoon). Air-fry for eighteen minutes. Shake and cook for six more minutes, then sprinkle with pepper and salt.
- Stir and melt together vegan butter, soy milk, and vegan cheddar until creamy.
- Serve fries smothered with cheese sauce and topped with chili, jalapeno rings, cilantro, and onion.

Saucy Onion Rings

Nutritional Facts: Calories 174 Fat 5.0 g Protein 7.0 g Carbohydrates 25.0 g

Prep Time: 15 min **Cook time:** 40 min

Servings: 4

Ingredients:

- Garlic powder (1/4 teaspoon)
- Paprika, smoked (1 teaspoon)
- Panko breadcrumbs, whole wheat (1 cup)
- Mayonnaise, canola (2 tablespoons)
- Egg, large (1 piece)
- Sweet onion, 10-ounce, sliced into half-inch-thick rings (1 piece)
- Mustard, Dijon (1 teaspoon)
- Flour, all purpose (1/2 cup)
- Salt, kosher, divided (1/2 teaspoon)
- Water (1 tablespoon)
- Greek yogurt, low fat, plain (1/4 cup)
- Ketchup (1 tablespoon)
- Paprika (1/4 teaspoon)
- Cooking spray

Directions:

- Combine flour, salt (1/4 teaspoon), and smoked paprika.
- Beat egg with water.
- Mix panko with salt (1/4 teaspoon).
- Dip onion rings in flour, then coat with egg mixture and cover with panko mixture. Mist cooking spray all over onion rings.
- Air-fry for five minutes on each side.
- Combine mayonnaise, mustard, paprika, garlic powder, ketchup, and yogurt.
- Serve onion rings with sauce.

Desserts

Chocolate Banana Packets

Nutritional Facts: Calories 270 Fat 7.0 g Protein 2.0 g Carbohydrates 50.0 g

Prep Time: 5 min *Cook time:* 15 min

Servings: 1

Ingredients:

- Miniature marshmallows (2 tablespoons)
- Cereal, cinnamon, crunchy, slightly crushed (2 tablespoons)
- Banana, peeled (1 piece)
- Chocolate chips, semi sweet (2 tablespoons)

Directions:

- Preheat air fryer to 390 degrees Fahrenheit.
- Slightly open banana by cutting lengthwise. Place on sheet of foil.
- Fill sliced banana with chocolate chips and marshmallows. Close foil packet.
- Air-fry for fifteen to twenty minutes.
- Open packet and top banana with crushed cereal.

Creamy Strawberry Mini Wraps

Nutritional Facts: Calories 190 Fat 4.5 g Protein 1.0 g Carbohydrates 22.0 g

Prep Time: 10 min *Cook time:* 15 min

Servings: 12

Ingredients:

- Cream cheese, softened (4 ounces)
- Strawberry jam (12 teaspoons)
- Pie crust, refrigerated (1 box)
- Powdered sugar (1/3 cup)

Directions:

- Preheat air fryer to 350 degrees Fahrenheit.
- Roll out pie crusts and cut out 12 squares.
- Beat together powdered sugar and cream cheese.
- Shape each dough square into a diamond before filling with cream cheese mixture (1 tablespoon). Top each with strawberry jam (1 teaspoon) and cover with dough sides.
- Place mini wraps on baking sheet and air-fry for fifteen minutes.

Heavenly Butter Cake Bars

Nutritional Facts: Calories 298.4 Fat 15.3 g Protein 2.8 g Carbohydrates 38.6 g

Prep Time: 15 min *Cook time:* 35 min

Servings: 12

Ingredients:

- Butter, melted (1/2 cup)
- Cream cheese (8 ounces)
- Vanilla (1 teaspoon)
- Cake mix, super moist, French vanilla (15 ¼ ounces)
- Eggs (3 pieces)
- Powdered sugar (1 pound)

Directions:

- Preheat air fryer to 325 degrees Fahrenheit.
- Use parchment to line baking dish.
- Combine cake mix with egg and melted butter to form soft dough. Press into baking dish.
- Beat together 2 eggs, cream cheese, vanilla, and sugar. Spread on top of cake mix layer.
- Air-fry for forty-five minutes. Let cool before slicing.

Tasty Shortbread Cookies

Nutritional Facts: Calories 70 Fat 4.0 g Protein 0 g Carbohydrates 7.0 g

Prep Time: 25 min *Cook time:* 1 hr 5 min

Servings: 4

Ingredients:

- Powdered sugar (3/4 cup)
- Flour, all purpose (2 ½ cups)
- Butter, softened (1 cup)
- Vanilla (1 teaspoon)

Directions:

- Preheat air fryer to 325 degrees Fahrenheit.
- Combine butter, vanilla and powdered sugar with flour to form a soft dough.
- Roll out dough and cut out 4 circles. Place on cookie sheet.
- Air-fry for fourteen to sixteen minutes.

Air-Fried Mini Pies

Nutritional Facts: Calories 196.3 Fat 8.4 g Protein 0.7 g Carbohydrates 29.9 g

Prep Time: 20 min *Cook time:* 55 min

Servings: 12

Ingredients:

- Pie filling (4 cups)
- Pie crusts, refrigerated (2 packages)
- Egg, whisked (1 piece)

Directions:

- Preheat air fryer to 325 degrees Fahrenheit.
- Mist cooking spray onto 12 muffin cups.
- Roll out pie crust and cut out twelve 4-inch circles. Press each onto bottom of a muffin cup. Cut remaining dough into thin strips.
- Add pie filling (1/4 cup) to each dough cup. Cover each with dough strips laid in a lattice pattern.
- Brush whisked egg on tops of pies and air-fry for thirty to forty minutes.

Pumpkin Pie Minis

Nutritional Facts: Calories 180 Fat 9.0 g Protein 1.0 g Carbohydrates 25.0 g

Prep Time: 25 min *Cook time:* 20 min

Servings: 12

Ingredients:

- Nutmeg (1/4 teaspoon)
- Brown sugar (3/8 cup)
- Pumpkin puree (1 cup)
- Cinnamon (1/2 teaspoon)
- Heavy cream (1 tablespoon)
- Egg, large (1 piece)
- Pie crust, refrigerated (1 package)

Directions:

- Preheat air fryer to 325 degrees Fahrenheit.
- Combine pumpkin, heavy cream, spices, and brown sugar.
- Unroll dough pieces and cut out twenty-four 2.5-inch circles. Place 12 circles on sheet of parchment. Top each with pie filling (1 tablespoon) and cover with another circle. Press to seal and brush all mini pies with whisked egg (1 piece). Dust all over with mixture of cinnamon and sugar.
- Air-fry for twenty minutes.

Mouthwatering Walnut Apple Pie Bites

Nutritional Facts: Calories 49.7 Fat 3.75 g Protein 0.6 g Carbohydrates 7.6 g

Prep Time: 10 min *Cook time:* 15 min

Servings: 8

Ingredients:

- Brown sugar (4 tablespoons)
- Butter, melted (1 tablespoon)
- Apple, tart juicy, red, washed, sliced into 8 portions, skin on (1 piece)
- Cinnamon (3 teaspoons)
- Crescent rolls, refrigerated (1 can)
- Walnuts, chopped finely (1 ounce)

Directions:

- Preheat air fryer to 325 degrees Fahrenheit.
- Roll out crescent rolls onto baking sheet misted with cooking spray.
- Brush melted butter on rolls before sprinkling with cinnamon and brown sugar. Add ¾ of finely chopped walnuts on top; press gently to adhere. Top each of wide ends with a slice of apple, then roll up. Brush melted butter on top of rolls before sprinkling with cinnamon and remaining ¼ of finely chopped walnuts.
- Air-fry for fifteen minutes.

Gooey Apple Pie Cookies

Nutritional Facts: Calories 211.8 Fat 4.5 g Protein 1.1 g Carbohydrates 44.2 g

Prep Time: 15 min *Cook time:* 20 min

Servings: 12

Ingredients:

- Egg, slightly beaten (1 piece)
- Caramel sauce (1 jar)
- Flour, all purpose (2 tablespoons)
- Pie crusts, refrigerated (1 package)
- Apple pie filling (1 can)
- Cinnamon sugar (3 tablespoons)

Directions:

- Preheat air fryer to 325 degrees Fahrenheit.
- Roll out dough and spread thinly with caramel sauce. Chop up apple pie filling and spread over caramel sauce. Cover with strips from other rolled out dough, laid to form a lattice pattern. Cut out 3-inch cookies and arrange on baking sheet.
- Air-fry for twenty to twenty-five minutes.

Apple Pie with Cinnamon Roll Crust

Nutritional Facts: Calories 255 Fat 10.0 g Protein 1.5 g Carbohydrates 39.0 g

Prep Time: 15 min *Cook time:* 55 min

Servings: 16

Ingredients:

Crust:

- Butter, unsalted, melted (1 tablespoon)
- Egg, beaten (1 piece) + water (1 teaspoon)—to make egg wash
- Pie crust, refrigerated (1 package)
- Cinnamon, ground (2 teaspoons)

Pie:

- Butter, unsalted, at room temp. (1 stick)
- Apples, Granny Smith, small, peeled, cored, sliced thinly (7 pieces)
- Sugar, light brown (1 cup)
- Flour, all purpose, unbleached (1 cup)
- Granulated sugar

Icing:

- Vanilla (1/4 teaspoon)
- Milk (2 teaspoons)
- Powdered sugar (1/2 cup)
- Cinnamon, ground (1/4 teaspoon)

Directions:

- Preheat air fryer to 375 degrees Fahrenheit.
- Unroll pie crust; brush top with butter before sprinkling with cinnamon. Roll up and slice into half-inch rounds.
- Press mini rolls into pie plate and brush tops with egg wash. Top with sliced apples. Cover with crumbly mixture of flour, brown sugar, and butter. Sprinkle with granulated sugar.
- Air-fry for forty to forty-five minutes.
- Finish by icing with whisked mixture milk, powdered sugar, cinnamon, and vanilla.

Sugar Cookie Cake

Nutritional Facts: Calories 295 Fat 15.5 g Protein 4.0 g Carbohydrates 35.0 g

Prep Time: 5 min *Cook time:* 35 min

Servings: 24

Ingredients:

- Condensed milk, sweetened (14 ounces)
- Cinnamon, ground (1 teaspoon)
- Butter, salted, melted (3/4 cup)
- Cookie butter (14 ounces)
- Eggs (3 pieces)
- Sugar cookie mix, prepared (17 ½ ounces)

Directions:

- Preheat air fryer to 325 degrees Fahrenheit. Mist cooking spray onto baking dish.
- Combine cookie butter with eggs, cinnamon, and condensed milk. Spread on baking dish and top with even layer of fry cookie mix. Drizzle melted butter on top and air-fry for thirty-five minutes.
- Let cool before slicing and serving.

Accessory #5 – Heat Resistant Tongs

Most food cooked in the Air Fryer will need to be flipped halfway through. Having a set of quality tongs is helpful. What better than a stainless steel silicone tong that's perfectly designed to help you turn over the food and prevent your hands from being burnt. The below tong does just that.

For more information about this accessory (and others that might interest you) go to:

www.MillenniumPublishingLimited.com > Barbara Trisler > Air Fryer Accessories

Conclusion

I hope this book was able to help you to understand the benefits of an Air Fryer and the basics on how to use it. The next step is to plan your meals and gather the ingredients. This appliance is easy to use and you will eventually get the hang of the process. Once you have tried several recipes, you can already start tweaking the ingredients to create variations or start making your own.

Enjoy the process of preparing your meals in a healthier way using this innovation when it comes to cooking.

The End

Thank you very much for taking the time to read this book. I tried my best to cover as many air fryer recipes as possible. If you found it useful please let me know by leaving a review on Amazon! Your support really does make a difference and I read all the reviews personally so can I understand what my readers particularly enjoyed and then feature more of that in future books.

I also pride myself on giving my readers the best information out there, being super responsive to them and providing the best customer service. If you feel I have fallen short of this standard in any way, please kindly email me at **BarbaraTrisler@yahoo.com** so I can get a chance to make it right to you.

I wish you all the best!

Index

How To Get The Bonus Recipe Image Booklet

1. Go to www.MillenniumPublishingLimited.com

2. Navigate to the tab labeled "Barbara Trisler" (hover over it)

3. Click on "Recipe Nutritional Fact Scorecard"

4. Specify where you want to receive the bonus nutritional fact scorecard & the recipe image booklet